Intermittent Fasting for Women

Discover scientific methods to burn fat in a guided and proven way + a 3-week diet plan to reset your metabolism and detoxify your body naturally and safely.

Elisabeth Holland

Table of contents

Introduction

Overweightness is widespread in most countries around the world. In fact, it has spread everywhere, and people are getting more and more obese because of their unhealthy way of living. The first reason is our eating habits.

Too many people are eating junk foods, processed foods, white flour products, etc. All of these foods can cause high blood sugar levels, which in turn can lead to fat buildup and decreased insulin sensitivity. The second reason is the sedentary lifestyle. Many manual operations have become easier and less demanding. Do you have to go to work for 20 minutes in the morning? You will drive instead of taking a walk. Do you need to go to the third floor of an office building? You will be using elevators instead of stairs, right?

Avoid all of these calorie-consuming activities and replace them with light alternatives. As a result, people gain weight. Watching TV is a lot easier than walking with a packet of potato chips. Drinking a bottle of Coca-Cola is much better than eating raw healthy food. Drink apple juice and clean water. All of these little actions are important. To make the problem worse, only the unhealthy food in the US groceries alone is generally cheaper than healthy and nutritious foods. You bought junk food but had a hard time paying for "really healthy organic food".

This is one of the reasons low-income families are the hardest hit by obesity. In fact, obesity is so severe that people can use this method to lose weight even if the diet is not healthy. Intermittent Fasting, unlike diets like the keto diet or the paleo diet, is a unique method that focuses on mealtimes rather than food intake. If you're trying to lose weight or can't control your appetite, the IF diet is your real answer.

Take a look at your abs, and see if you can burn the last layer of belly fat? The intermittent name fasting is everywhere. In fact, it is one of the most effective and outstanding ways to lose weight, and it is an amazing solution for most people who try to lose weight and feel healthy. It's very simple and sturdy, and it reflects nature and common sense. Most importantly, it works, and the results show almost like magic.

This book is called "Intermittent Fasting for Women," and it can change the life of any woman. This guide is divided into two parts, divided into Intermittent Fasting and an Introduction to Healthy Recipes. Get ready because it's going to be a great moment for all women in the world!

Thanks for your preference.

I wish you a pleasant reading and, if you like this book, write a review, please. I'll be grateful.

PART 1

What is Intermittent Fasting (IF)

Intermittent Fasting is the fad in fitness, health and weight reduction circles with thoughts making it huge in practice. It's famous as it works stunningly. IF is a nutrients cycle, a manner of consuming, and it's focusing on the way you devour the meals, now no longer what to devour. Try now; wait no longer if you want to stray a long way from this basis in case you count to gain the entire sweets of IF.

There are numerous varieties of intermittent fasting. This chapter will spotlight a number of the famous ones and suggest the very best type to observe to make certain that your existence does now no longer emerge as miserable.

Intermittent Fasting may be damaged down into two segments:

- Fasting window
- Eating window

You will now no longer be allowed to devour any meals. You need to drink a lot of water too. No energy has to be spent in the course of the fasting window. During the consuming window, you may be allowed to devour and could want to devour all of your energy for the day in the course of this window. Eat excessive fibre foods, including nuts, beans, culmination and vegetables, and excessive protein foods, together with meat, fish, tofu, or nuts, in the course of your consuming window. Chewing excessive fibre gummies can additionally help, so keep that in your thoughts too.

Intermittent fasting does not make a problem what you eat. The food plan is secondary, and it's focusing extra on how and whilst you want to eat, not what to eat, what virtually subjects is what you have to be compliant in the course of the fasting period. This is the frame that will make use of its fat cells for energy.

When you're at a caloric deficit, and also you integrate it with intermittent fasting, your fats go to soften off quicker than what you ever concept possible. Let's take a look at one easy example:

If you've got got an eight-hour consuming window and a sixteen-hour fasting window, you may want to devour all of your energy for the day in the course of the eight hours. It means that your frame will now no longer have to move into "hunger mode" due to the fact you are consuming and ingesting energy. You're simply doing it within a quick span of time. So, assuming you devour all of your energy in the course of the eight hours, approximately three to four hours after your remaining meal, the meals you ate might have been digested. From here, approximately 12 hours left to head earlier than your subsequent meal, considering that you're on a sixteen-hour frame. Your frame will now no longer have any extra meals to apply as body fuel.

That is whilst it's going to use the insulin and fats reserves for energy. It doesn't depend on case you're sleeping or not, and your frame will nonetheless be burning energy for all of the special physical strategies, including restoring and maintenance. These foods might be coming out of your saved fats. This is what makes IF so fantastic. Like Leonardo da Vinci said, "Simplicity is the ultimate sophistication". Intermittent fasting is extraordinarily easy in concept.

It doesn't contain detoxification, low carbs, ketogenic dieting, etc. None of that is an issue. All you need to do is to eat and fast, that's it. It doesn't get any simpler.

Now let's have a take a look at the way it got here approximately.

Where does IF Originate from?

There isn't any unique region from which IF originated. In reality, it's focusing primarily on the food-based manner our ancestors ate. In the past, meals have changed into scarce. If our ancestor wanted to eat, they needed to hunt. On days whilst we controlled our meals and searching for it changed into successful activity, there feast come out. As the pickings have been narrowed down and there haven't been meals, you'd move hungry. This might be a way to fasting. The handiest distinction is that there wasn't a preference within the past.

Because of this way of consuming and fasting, our ancestors have seldom been overweight. They additionally led a lot of extra energetic lives considering that there changed into no generation to help them. So, we are able to count on to sure knowledge that the human frame instinctively adapts to intermittent fasting. We also additionally have evolved technologically. However, in terms of our physiology, we're quite a lot similar to our ancestors in both eating and fasting.

Is Intermittent Fasting Safe Enough?

In reality, it'll be tremendously beneficial. Studies have proven that many folks that began out intermittent fasting achieved fitness advantages, including accelerated fats burning and a higher metabolic rate. Their blood pressure, cholesterol degrees and blood sugar level decrease dramatically.

If you're involved properly, IF will overwin your fears. Everybody needs to undergo fasting days after they sleep. If you want to sleep around eight hours, you may input your fasted period. The foremost reason that many humans no longer revel in the advantages of this fasting period is because of the reality that older people get much less than eight hours of sleep. Furthermore, humans eat earlier than going to bed.

So, whilst they're consuming the food, the meals are being digested. The frame doesn't get a treatment during the fasting period for too long. The second reason is that they wake up, have breakfast and begin consuming other foods at some stage in the day. There could be very little time for the frame to faucet into its fat cells. As we have mentioned previously, people with diabetes, gastric issues, or similar problems have to see a doctor earlier than an intermittent fasting period. Your doctor will for sure nicely advise you in case you have to stop with it immediately.

Why is Intermittent Fasting so popular?

The reality of the problem is that you have to examine your food consuming habits, your eating patterns, your task requirements, etc. You have to tailor the way of healthy living for you. If you figure out your night period, you can't eat via the nighttime due to the fact you may be hungry. So, you have to encompass your eating hours into your fasting window and perhaps begin your consuming window 6 hours after waking up.

Of course, that is assuming that you undertake the primary type of intermittent fasting. You may additionally have social activities, etc., that might also additionally make your intermittent fasting period difficult for you. Sooner or later, your fasting will cramp your social existence. Once again, you may want to hang out around it.

Ultimately, you have to pick a way that you suppose will support you. From here, you will no longer get over-formidable or overestimate your will-strength and choose to head for the 24 hours period on the primary day. It can be really problematic for older people. You may turn it out to be giving up and hard-consuming. Later on, you can additionally enjoy emotions of guilt and can experience your failures. This is in which older humans throw withinside the towel. They suppose they have got failed, whilst in reality, they simply set unreasonable goals. The key to achievement is to make measurable progress with affordable goals.

Why start IF, advantages and disadvantages

You may want to begin a temporary fasting lifestyle, but you may be concerned about safety. After all, not all diets are suitable for everyone. Adequate nutrition is a key factor in safe and successful weight loss. Vitamins and proteins are important part and without them, you could get sick. With too few calories and too restrictive eating habits, you may not be getting enough nutrients results. This can lead to medical problems. The good news is that intermittent fasting seems like a safe way to eat for most people.

However, there are some cases when intermittent fasting should be avoided. Most people who embark on this lifestyle hope to lose weight and maintain a healthy weight. Why do people need to start intermittent fasting? Here we're going over some pros and cons, so pay close attention to them:

ADVANTAGES

1. Reduce body fat quickly and safely.

This is the main reason that most people will investigate the IF approach to dieting as long as you take your fast days serious. If you eat much these days, you are obviously missing the point. Recent research from the University of Illinois showed that the following calorie-reduction plans lost significantly more fat on day two than those who ate normally and followed the same exercise protocols. Unfortunately, most of the time, they lag far behind the actual top of health and nutrition.

2. Easy manage what you eat

The following innovative benefit of IF is how easy it is to follow and manage. We've already mentioned it in this eBook, but it's really worth repeating. Anyone who has counted carbohydrates on a ketogenic diet, for example, or the many other diets, will be quick to agree. Once you have calculated in your head what your 500 or 600 calories will look like on the day of fasting, you are good to go. No calculators or complications needed.

3. Improved Mental Function

Reducing weekly calories leads to greater focus, better memory, and other improved cognitive functions, according to research by Mark Mattson for The Lancet. These effects can even translate into fighting Alzheimer's disease and other similar health problems.

4. Improving Insulin Levels

One of the reasons many people pack and find it so difficult to lose body fat is their runaway insulin levels. The IF approach optimizes insulin levels for healthy fat loss and increases the amount of fat that has already been reduced by the calorie reduction and increased metabolism. On fast days, small meals and the lack of constant eating or grazing, free a shocking amount of time and energy. The IF diet is packed with physical, mental and even social benefits, and it is hard to think of anything but a minor inconvenience or two and only for those who lack a desire to "lose weight".

This really is a life changing method for the better life many people need to start on IF, but there are also people who should avoid taking IF. They are:

- Children because of their growth and physical development.
- Pregnant and diabetics due to side effects on blood sugar and insulin
- Breastfeeding women due to their particular diet during pregnancy so that the baby develops properly.

Here are some problems that IF can cause in any consumer, which is why it is also billed as a disadvantage of IF.

DISADVANTAGES

The Problem of Being Slim and Healthy

While we are allowed and encouraged to eat freely and joyfully on the fasting days, it doesn't mean we have to eat whole like a wolverine. So, if you're not losing weight the way you'd like and eating endless fries, ice cream, and candy on your fasting days, adjust your diet and eat healthier calories or less every other day.

They also did not harm his body in any way. If you are experiencing a lot of stress and discomfort every other day because you are hungry, it is time to gain more control over your mind. It does this by developing your willpower, following things like this diet even if you'd rather not, and focusing on the end result you want. Be tough and get rewarded.

Types of IF

There are several different types of intermittent fasting. Usually, the differences will depend on the person creating the method. The fundamentals of an eating window and a fasting window will always apply. Bear in mind that it really doesn't matter which method you choose. All the different methods will reap rewards. You should pick one that you're comfortable with.

When the method you choose is easy for you to follow, the chances of you complying with it and staying the course will be much higher. Initially, if you're new to intermittent fasting, you will want to take it slow and have a longer eating window and a shorter fasting window. It will take about 2 weeks to a month for your body to adapt to your new way of eating. There is no doubt that you will most probably encounter resistance and cravings from your body.

This is par for the course. After all, most people are used to eating throughout their waking hours. Restricting your eating hours can be stressful in the beginning. Rest assured that with time, your body will adapt, and you will be surprised to see that your appetite has decreased. You will also feel more alert, energetic and slimmer as you progress.

Now let's look at some of the intermittent fasting types:

1. 16:8 IF type

16:8 IF type is the best type of intermittent fasting to start with if you are a beginner. This is an eating plan which allows you to have 16 hours of fasting, then normal eating period of 8 hours of the day. This method is mostly used by people, and it's well known among the IF consumers.

2. 24-Hours Intermittent Fasting

The 2nd method of intermittent fasting is known as Eat Stop Eat and was created by Brad Pilon. His program is actually an online bestseller. The rules of the fast are pretty simple. You will fast for 24 hours twice or thrice a week. On days when you're not fasting, you may eat what you want without worry. In this manner, your overall consumption of calories for the week will be less and you will lose weight. Since you are allowed to eat whatever, you want to eat during the eating window, you will not be deprived of your favorite foods.

This can be a relief to many people who fear giving up the foods they love. However, the 24-hour break from eating can be extremely difficult for many people. So, as mentioned earlier, you may follow Martin's method and work your way up.

3. 20:4 Fasting

The 3rd IF type is known as the Warrior Diet and it was created by Ori Hofmekeler. This is a much more severe method that Martin's one. The rules state that you'll need to fast for 20 hours a day and only eat 1 large meal every night. This is supposedly what our ancestors may have done. While it's anyone's guess as to whether our ancestors really ate in this manner, the fact remains that Ori's method is highly effective. Many people who adopted his method have seen vast benefits to their health.

Initially, when you're starting out, you might not want to use Ori's method. It would be a better idea to start off with Marin's method and gradually reduce your eating window over time till you are able to fast for 20 hours without discomfort. Don't jump into the deep end of the pool and struggle with a 20 hour fast. You should also know that Ori's method does allow a few small meals during the fasting window. However, there are rules as to what you can eat and cannot eat. So, you will need to watch your diet and stick to the approved food list. This is definitely one of the stricter methods of IF.

4. 5:2 Fasting

This popular form of intermittent fasting involves eating normally for five days every week. For the remaining two days, calories should be restricted to 500 – 600. Sometimes called the Fast Diet, this way of eating was made popular by Michael Mosley, a journalist. Women are recommended to eat 500 calories on their fasting days. Men can have 600 calories on their fast days. You can pick your two favourite days for fasting, and you can do it on your own terms. Keep in mind that you need to intake up to 500 calories; people often take 200 or 300 on their fasting days.

5. 36-Hour Fasting

The 36-hour fast plan means you'll be fasting for a full day. Unlike the Eat-Stop-Eat method, you won't be eating something every calendar day. If, for example, you finish dinner at 7 p.m. on day one, you skip all your meals on day two. You won't eat your next meal until day three at 7 a.m. This equals a 36-hour fast. There is some evidence to suggest this kind of fasting period can produce a quicker result. It may also be beneficial for diabetics. It may also be more problematic, though, since you'll be going for extended periods without food.

6. Alternate Day Fasting (ADF)

This way of fasting means that you fast for a full 24 hours every alternate day. Some versions of this IF diet allow you to eat up to 500 calories on a fast day. Others only allow you to have calorie-free beverages. This isn't the best option for any newcomers to intermittent fasting. You go to bed feeling hungry several nights each week. This is hard to maintain in the long term.

7. Extended Fasts

Following the 16:8 or Eat-Stop-Eat method is quite simple. Some people, though, are keen to push the benefits of intermittent fasting to the limit. They prefer to do a 42-hour fast. This involves eating dinner on day 1, say at 6 p.m. All meals would be skipped on the next day. On day 3, you would then eat your breakfast at noon. This would be a total fasting time of 42 hours.

If you try this way of eating, you shouldn't restrict your calorie intake during your eating window. It's technically possible to extend fasts for longer periods of time. In fact, the world record stands at 382 days. Of course, that isn't recommended! Some people do try 7 to 14 day fasts due to the theoretical benefits they are said to provide. Some people say that a seven-day fast can help prevent cancer. Others say that longer fasts promote mental clarity. These benefits are unproven and are theoretical. It's probably best, therefore, to stick to one of the tried and tested IF plans outlined above.

Keep in mind all of these types before you start with IF. Choose the most acceptable for you and do it on the most proper way.

Food to eat and to avoid

If you follow an IF lifestyle there are no restrictions on what you can eat in your feeding window. This is why it is so different from other diets. You are not limited to specific amounts or types of food. However, it is wise to remember that you still need to make healthy choices. If you overdo it on a regular basis, you won't see the benefits of IF. The best solution is a balanced diet in your eating window. This will help you maintain your energy levels while losing weight at the same time. Nutrient-rich foods like seeds, beans, nuts, whole grains, vegetables, and fruits are good choices. You also eat a lot of lean protein.

There are foods that are especially useful when following the IF diet:

Avocados - Yes, they are high in calories. However, they are full of monounsaturated fats. That makes them very satisfying. Adding half an avocado to your meal will make you feel a lot fuller.

Fish - must treat at least 8 ounces of fish a week. Fish is full of protein, healthy fats, and vitamin D. It's good for your brain health too.

Vegetables - are an important part of the IF diet.

There are many vegetables that are great to eat when starting or planning to begin the IF diet:

- Kale
- Spinach
- Swiss chard
- Cabbage
- Collard Greens

Cruciferous vegetables: foods like cauliflower, Brussels sprouts, and broccoli are good choices. They're full of fibre to help prevent constipation and make you feel fuller. ·

Potatoes - Many people worry that potatoes are bad for you, but they are very satisfying and will keep you satisfied for longer.

Legumes and Beans: Although they are carbohydrates, they are low in calories and give you lots of energy. packed with protein and fiber.

Probiotics: When you eat foods rich in probiotics like sauerkraut, kefir, and kombucha, your gut will stay happy. This will help you avoid stomach problems as you adjust to this diet.

Berries - Strawberries, blueberries, and others are filled with nutrients like vitamin C. They're also high in flavonoids, which are known to stimulate weight loss.

Eggs: Each egg contains 6 grams of protein. Eggs are easy and quick to cook and will keep you feeling full.

Nuts: Nuts are high in calories. However, they are full of polyunsaturated fats that will help you feel full.

Full grain: Whole grains are carbohydrates too! However, they are filled with protein and fiber. You don't have to overeat to feel full longer. One study even showed that consuming whole grains can boost your metabolism. These are the foods that you will need to practice.

When will it start with IF?

Since you must consume certain foods, there are also foods that you should avoid when starting your IF diet regardless of your age. These foods, which are dangerous to your diet and are caloric, high in sugar and fat. They won't fill your body after fasting, and they can even make you hungrier. They also provide a very low level of good nutritional facts for your body.

Here's an explanation for this too:

- Unhealthy chips.
- Microwave popcorn
- You should also watch out for foods rich in sugar.

The added sugars in processed foods and beverages are filled with dangerous amounts of sweet, empty calories, which is really bad for your diet and your desired results. It's the opposite of your end goals when you're in IF. They increase your feeling of hunger than ultrafast sugar processing.

Sugary foods to avoid include:

- Barbecue sauce and ketchup.

- Fruit juice.
- Cookies
- Sugary cereals and granola.
- Candy
- Cakes

Mistakes to avoid during IF

People make different mistakes when they start with IF. Below is a list of the most common mistakes many people make. Hence, all of these mistakes must be avoided in order to successfully perform intermittent fasting.

1. Pigging

People want to be in the focus on the subject of being slim and healthy. While we can and may eat freely and happily on vacation, this does not mean that we have the full permision to eat a glutton. So, if you're not losing weight the way you'd like and eating endless fries, ice cream, and candy on your vacation, adjust your diet and eat healthier.

2. Fear of Starving All Day

Nobody starved to death by eating 500 calories or less every other day. They also did not harm his body in any way. So, if you are experiencing a lot of stress and discomfort every other day because you are hungry, it is time to gain more control over your mind. It does this by developing your willpower, following things like this diet even if you'd rather not, and focusing on the end result you want. Be tough and you will be rewarded.

3. Eating Too Much On Your Fasting Days

Let's not play games, 500 calories or less means 500 calories or less. If you eat cleanly while on vacation and still don't lose weight, it likely means that you overeat on starvation days. Calorie counting to make sure you have 500 calories or less.

4. Reduce Your Activity

It is tempting for some to slow down their activities during fasting days. Don't fall for it. In fact, with a bit of experience with festivals, you will find that hunger days release more energy, and you need to make an effort to be even more active. Doing more is almost always better than doing nothing.

5. Hanging out with wrong people

Being with people who disregard your dieting efforts, as well as close friends and family, who would it be? It's hard to avoid, it's a disappointment to be around people who are trying to speak negatively about you or who are trying to keep you from achieving your IF goals.

Again, the diet is 90% mental, so don't let other people mess with your mental game. It's annoying, defeatist, and unnecessary! Beginner mistakes are easy to avoid, and if you stumble it's okay just keep going. The IF diet was designed to be effective, open, and easy to use. A little self reflection and you will quickly be back on track and take over the body and life of your dreams! For older women, Pilates is a good idea for a day or an easy walk. The key is to get more exercise and challenge yourself. It is a difficult habit to get across, but very easy to lose. Intermittent fasting will help you lose weight and lose weight.

Exercise not only speeds up the process, it also prevents fat in the long run. It is a fact that most people can lose weight, but often they cannot keep the weight off for long. You have days to exercise and days to rest. Never skip a day of training because you are out of the mood. Once you do, you will find that you don't have that mood to train the next day and before you know it, you stopped training for 3 weeks. Now you have to keep fighting to get started. If you don't want to lose momentum, don't stop. Short rest days of 1 day are sufficient. If you don't exercise excessively, 1 rest day every three days is enough to give your body a break. Now that you know what the most common mistakes are, you can make them, avoid them and be successful with intermittent fasting. Save all of the above information and examples and keep up to date on all IF things.

Autophagy

Autophagy is a term which means "eat-yourself", but rest assured, this is a good thing. Autophagy is the method your body uses to cleanse damaged cells and toxins, helping you regenerate newer, healthier cells. Over time, our cells accumulate a multitude of dead organelles, damaged proteins, and oxidized particles that hinder the body's internal functions.

This accelerates the effects of aging and age-related diseases because cells cannot divide and function normally. This lysosome-dependent cell regeneration process is critical to your overall health. Indeed, autophagy dysfunction has been linked to several neurodegenerative diseases, including Alzheimer's disease. Since many of our cells, like those in the brain, have to last a lifetime, the body has developed a unique method to rid itself of these defective parts and to defend itself naturally against disease.

Think of your body as a kitchen. After you've prepared a meal, clean the counter and throw it away. Leftovers and recycle some of the food. The next day you have a clean kitchen. This is autophagy that does its job on your body and gets it right. Now imagine the same scenario, but you are older and inefficient. After you've prepared the food, leave leftovers on the counter. Some are thrown away, and some are not. Leftovers remain on the counter, in the garbage and in the trash.

You never make it out of the garbage can door, and toxic waste builds up in your kitchen. There is fermented food on the floor and all kinds of foul smells blowing through the door. Because of the onslaught of pollutants and toxins, you have a scenario similar to autophagy, which doesn't work as well as it should. Usually, the autophagy hums softly behind the scenes Maintenance mode plays a role in how your body responds to periods of stress, maintains balance, and regulates cell function. Plus, you can't forget about your mitochondrial health.

Through a process called mitophagy, the excess of mitochondria is broken down autophagy. Evidence that triggering autophagy will slow the aging process, reduce inflammation, and improve your overall performance. To help your body resist disease and maintain longevity, there are ways you can naturally increase your autophagy response (more on that later).

We are only just beginning to understand how autophagy works in the body, and what we know so far is largely based on rodent studies. We are not human, but the evidence is overwhelming. Autophagy is said to:

- Control inflammation, slow the aging process, and protect against neurodegenerative diseases.
- Work against infections and support immunity.
- Help live longer by improving cells' metabolic fitness by removing damaged organelles and proteins.

How to get started with Intermittent Fasting

If you are convinced of the benefits of intermittent fasting, you need to know how to get started. After all, embarking on a new regime can be difficult. So what's the best way to get started? Thank you for your time to read this eBook and we really hope you found it useful and insightful. We have no doubt that when you focus on the IF diet, achieve your weight loss goals, and more. When do you plan to start? If you have only hesitated, you may experience the greatest enemy of attaining your dream body of all: what is known as procrastination.

Let's go over some tips that can help you slaughter this beast and start your own transformation story:

1. Just Do It

The IF Diet doesn't require any specific foods, supplements, or information beyond this e-book to be good work and opportunity. So, what are you waiting for? Say YES now. The only thing stopping you is your own indolence. Eliminate any thoughts from tomorrow or next week. Make another decision and start now.

2. Eliminate your excuses

Do you have recurring excuses why you can't start a temporary fast today? Say these excuses out loud so you can hear how ridiculously counterproductive they are. If you still have doubts, write them down and burn them as you break free of limiting beliefs.

3. Look yourself at a mirror

If you are fat, the mirror and lack of clothes do not lie. Remind yourself that your body will not get more comfortable until you first make a decision to change it and then take steps to support that decision. This measure consists in adopting the IF diet wisely. If not, it likely looks the same, if not worse, than in the mirror for the coming days, weeks, months, and years. That might sound harsh, but a hard truth is much better than a nice lie.

4. Stop wasting time.

Do you need that much social networking, television, or gaming? Video games when your body is not where you want it to be? Do you put the light and the distracting before the vital and important? If yes, why? Break the trance, don't waste any more time and build your new you now!

5. Write down your goals clearly and in details.

As possible, do it as soon as possible because there is something magical about the written word, especially when it comes to setting and achieving goals. That magic is even more pronounced when the written words are yours. Write down and read through your goals, big and small, and accept YES as a means to get you in the direction you need to go. There is no living success trainer or sports psychologist to argue with. against this advice! You shouldn't either.

Are you psychological when dealing with IF? We knew it would be you. This could be a day when you look back decades and say, "That's where I made serious life-improving changes! The things this lifestyle offers are so serious. We'd love it. Hear your success story, so stay You" Then you know what to eat in your dining room window. Can you consume during your Lent? The answer depends on how fast you are working.

If you follow the 5:2 diet, you can eat up to 500 to 600 calories on your fasting days. That is of course quite restrictive. You can maximize the amount you can eat by adding lots of low-calorie, nutrient-dense foods. Vegetables and fruits are staples on your fasting days. You can not eat any solid food at all. You also can't have a drink that has calories in it. Fortunately, however, there are plenty of drinks that you will need to keep hydrated. It is obvious that you need to have plenty of water in your fasting window and still water is fine. If you'd like, you can add a dash of lime or lemon for a little more flavor. You can also add more flavor with orange or cucumber slices. However, you cannot add an artificially sweetened enhancer.

These could harm your fast. Another good drink for your fasting is black coffee. It's calorie-free and doesn't affect your insulin. You can drink coffee or regular coffee, but you cannot add milk or sweeteners. If you want more flavor, try adding cinnamon or other spices. Some people say that black coffee could increase IF benefits. Caffeine can aid in ketone production. It can also help maintain healthy blood sugar levels over the long term.

Some people find this when they drink coffee while fasting have an upset stomach or racing heart. You may need to keep an eye on how you feel when you drink black coffee. If you are fasting for 24 hours or more, try vegetable or bone broth. Do not use diced or canned broth, because it's full of artificial preservatives and flavors that will harm your fast.

Exercises to do with the IF

As mentioned in this e-book, you should definitely exercise and move your body as much as possible. There are many benefits of exercise such as:

- Higher metabolism that helps you lose fat
- Releases endorphins that make you happier
- Prevents muscle wasting. If you don't use it, you will lose it.
- Improves blood circulation
- It prevents diseases that cause cognitive impairment
- Promotes Better Sleep
- Keeps Your Weight Under Control
- And Much More!

Moving from a sedentary to an active lifestyle can take a tremendous effort. The key here is making small daily improvements. If you haven't exercised in years, you can start with a 20-minute walk every day. Don't jump into a high-intensity workout overnight. Give your body time to adjust and recover. Start with low impact exercises like walking, cycling, and swimming. Then go on in strength training with light weights.

There is no need to train to exhaustion, though. What matters is that you get more exercise and get into the habit of exercising regularly. Over time, you can increase the intensity of your exercise and challenge yourself. Remember, it's okay to exercise on an empty stomach. However, it is preferable that you eat within 45 minutes of completing your workout.

So, you can exercise during your feeding period or start your feeding period after exercise. That sums it up pretty well. A clean diet, intermittent fasting ... and regular exercise are the three sides of the weight loss triangle. When you have all three components in place, you will lose weight, be healthier and fitter, and keep the extra pounds off. Whether you are doing it for weight loss or for other benefits, you will likely want to maximize your results.

Fortunately, there are a few things you can do to get the most of it. For anyone who has chosen IF, not just women over 50. There is some research showing that exercising on an empty stomach has additional benefits. There is an impact on muscle metabolism and biochemistry. This is related to insulin sensitivity and blood sugar levels. If you exercise while fasting, the stored carbohydrates will be used up. This means that you are burning more fat.

For the best result, eat protein after your workout and maintain your muscles. It will also better promote and resume the carbohydrate weight training within half an hour of your workout. It is recommended that you eat near an intense or modern workout session. You also need to drink a lot more water than usual to stay well hydrated. Coconut water can help with this a little lightheaded or dizzy if you exercise while fasting. When you experience this, take a break. It is important that you listen to your body. If you fast longer, look for gentle exercises like pilates, yoga, or walking.

Fat without making you feel bad. Not all workouts are timed to be the same. Some types of exercises tend to be. Muscles can be more tiring, and these may require a meal immediately after or a higher carbohydrate intake earlier in the day. Let's look at a few of these:

Cardio Exercise and HIIT

When done right, rapid cardio can be a great addition to your exercise plan. Depending on the type of exercise you are doing, you may not need to eat right after. If it is a high-intensity cardiovascular exercise that may have a strength-based component, we would like it to be closer to when they would break their fast. If you run slowly and steadily in the morning, you can wait a few hours after your workout to start eating. However, if this makes you feel weak and dizzy, try to eat immediately after your workout. When people have severe hypoglycemia and are fasting uncomfortably, it may take time to relieve strenuous cardiovascular exercise. To be able to achieve these fasting states gradually increase your vigorous exercise as your body learns to adapt to exercises on an empty stomach.

Strength Training

To gain muscle mass, it is important to consume large amounts of protein and complex carbohydrates before or immediately after training. Working to gain mass and strength, do this just before the break of the fast or in the feeding window, not at the end of the Feeding windows if they cannot be restored afterwards. If you do your weight training during the feeding window, your muscles will have enough fuel to do the job without collapsing. It really comes down to what makes you feel best.

Ask yourself what your training goals are. Do you want to feel during your workout and how do you really feel during your workout?

PART 2

3 WEEKS DIET PLAN

Following an easy 3-week meal plan to start is great way to get on the right track and become familiar with the IF guidelines. You will find that most of the foods on the plan are familiar and easy to find in your local grocery store. So, make you comfortable and start reading the 21-days diet meal list. Accept the challenge and be a better version of yourself.

1. DAY 1

- Servings - 1
- Cooking Time - 20-30 min

Breakfast

- Oatmeal with Pistachios and Currants

Lunch - Basil Chicken Wrap

- 1 tomato, sliced
- 1 medium tortilla
- 3 ounces cooked, chopped chicken breast
- ½ cup halved green grapes
- 1 t-spoon pecan pieces
- 1 t-spoon plain fat-free yogurt
- 1 cup fat-free milk or tea

Snack

- 1½ cups broccoli

Dinner

- Coconut Fish Stew

- **Nutritional facts:** Kcal - 834, carbs - 12g, protein - 51.4g, fat - 27.4g

2. DAY 2

- Servings 1
- Cooking Time - 30-40 min

Breakfast

- 1 light multigrain English muffin
- ½ cup sliced strawberries
- 1 t-spoon almond butter
- 1 t-spoon unsalted sunflower seeds
- 1 cup vanilla fat-free yogurt
- 1 cup apple juice

Lunch

- Crunchy Chicken Salad

Snack

- Thai Pork in Lettuce Wraps

Dinner - Grilled Pork Tenderloin

- 4 ounces grilled pork tenderloin rubbed with nutmeg
- 1 small baked potato
- 1 t-spoon fat-free plain yogurt
- 1 t-spoon sliced green onions Mixed green salad

- 2 cups green-leaf lettuce
- ½ cup halved cherry tomatoes
- ½ cup cucumber slices

Nutritional facts: Kcal - 1124, carbs - 17g, protein - 84.4g, fat - 32.4g

3. DAY 3

- Servings – 1 - Cooking Time - 20-30 min

Breakfast

- 1 medium peach
- 1 small whole-wheat pita with
- 2 t-spoons sodium-free peanut butter
- 1 cup fat-free milk
- Decaffeinated coffee or herbal tea

Lunch

- Simple tomato soup

Snack

- 2 plums
- 1 cup fat-free yogurt
- 1 t-spoon raw sunflower seeds

Dinner

- Egg Noodles
-

Nutritional facts: Kcal - 750, carbs - 15g, protein - 55.8g, fat - 19.4g

4. DAY 4

- Servings – 1 - Cooking Time - 30-40 min

Breakfast

- Egg Omelet

Lunch - Pasta Salad

- 1 small tomato, chopped
- 1 cup cooked whole-wheat or rice pasta
- ½ cup sliced mushrooms
- ½ yellow pepper, seeded and chopped
- ⅓ cup chopped red onion
- 2 t-spoons low-fat
- 1 cup fresh fruit juice

Snack

- ⅓ cup low-fat cottage cheese
- ½ cup blueberries
- 1 tablespoon pumpkin seeds

Dinner

- Roast Chicken

Nutritional facts: Kcal - 952, carbs - 13g, protein - 65.7g, fat - 23g

5. Day 5

- Servings - 2
- Cooking Time - 25-35 min

Breakfast - Strawberry Waffles

- 2 whole-grain waffles
- ¼ cup fat-free cottage cheese
- 2 t-spoons slivered almonds
- 1 cup sliced strawberries
- 1 cup herbal tea or coffee

Lunch - Crab Papaya Salad

- 3 ounces real crab meat
- 2 t-spoons chopped cilantro
- 1 large papaya, peeled, seeded and sliced into strips
- 2 cups baby spinach leaves
- ½ yellow pepper, seeded and chopped finely
- 3 thin slices of red onion
- 1 cup cherry tomatoes
- ½ cup cucumber slices
- 2 t-spoons red wine vinaigrette
- Herbal cold tea

Snack

- Baked Applesauce with Walnuts

Dinner

- Turkey and Black Beans

Nutritional facts: Kcal - 1246, carbs - 22g, protein - 53g, fat - 15g

6. Day 6

- Servings 1
- Cooking Time - 30-40 min

Breakfast

- ¾ cup cooked quinoa (cooked with 1.3 cup water and ½ cup skim milk)
- ½ cup unsweetened applesauce
- 2 t-spoons pecans
- ½ whole-wheat pita with 1 t-spoons almond or nut butter
- 1 banana
- Herbal tea

Lunch - Mushroom Burgers

- 1 large Portobello mushroom
- 1 whole-wheat burger bun
- 1 tablespoon goat cheese
- ½ small tomato sliced
- 1 slice red onion
- 2 Bibb lettuce leaves
- 1 cup baby carrots
- ¼ cup fat-free ranch dressing
- 1 cup skim milk

Snack

- Popcorns

Dinner - Spaghetti with Fresh Tomato Sauce

- 2 cups carrot noodles (strips of carrot made with a peeler) tossed with 2 large tomatoes, chopped
- ½ cup artichoke hearts, quartered
- 1 teaspoon chopped fresh basil
- 1 tablespoon grated Parmesan cheese
- Pinch red chili pepper flakes
- 2 cups chopped romaine
- 1 tablespoon low-fat Caesar dressing
- 1 cup melon, cubed
- Sparkling water or herbal iced tea

Nutritional facts: Kcal - 774, carbs - 15g, protein - 49.6g, fat - 25g

7. Day 7

- Servings – 2
- Cooking Time - 40-50 min

Breakfast

- 1 banana, sliced
- 1 cup bran flakes cereal
- 1 cup skim milk
- ½ cup sliced strawberries
- 1 t-spoon plain fat-free yogurt

Lunch - Greek Steak Pita Sandwiches

- 2 whole-wheat pitas
- 1 cup shredded romaine lettuce
- 1 small tomato
- ⅓ small red onion, peeled and sliced thinly
- 2 t-spoons low-fat, low-sodium feta cheese
- 2 cups cubed watermelon
- 1 cup skim milk or tea

Snack

- Healthy Chips

Dinner

- Chicken Breasts with Brown Rice

Nutritional facts: Kcal - 1266, carbs - 17g, protein - 27g, fat - 25g

8. Day 8

- Servings 1
- Cooking Time - 40-50 min

Breakfast - Peanut Butter Smoothie

- 1 banana
- ½ cup fat-free vanilla yogurt
- 2 t-spoon salt-free peanut butter
- 1 cup sliced strawberries
- ½ cup skim milk or tea

Lunch

- Kali Salad

Snack

- 1 cup vanilla fat-free, low-calorie yogurt
- 4 graham crackers

Dinner - Grilled Pork Tenderloin

- 4 ounces grilled pork tenderloin rubbed with nutmeg
- 1 small baked potato
- 1 t-spoon fat-free plain yogurt
- 1 t-spoon sliced green onions

- Mixed green salad
- 2 cups green-leaf lettuce
- ½ cup halved cherry tomatoes
- ½ cup cucumber slices

Nutritional facts: Kcal - 887, carbs - 42g, protein - 52.3g, fat - 12g

9. Day 9

- Servings – 1 - Cooking Time - 40-50 min

Breakfast

- Breakfast Hash

Lunch

- White Beans and Soup

Snack

- 1-ounce light cheese
- 1 cup baby carrots

Dinner - Chicken Soft Taco

- 1 multigrain tortilla
- ½ cup black beans
- 4 ounces cooked chopped chicken
- ½ cup shredded iceberg lettuce
- ½ ripe avocado, sliced
- ½ small tomato, chopped
- 1 cup unsweetened applesauce
- 1 healthy tea

Nutritional facts: Kcal - 812, carbs - 37g, protein - 49.6g, fat - 25g

10. Day 10

- Servings - 1
- Cooking Time - 40-50 min

Breakfast

- Fruit Filled Toast

Lunch

- White Bean and Soup

Snack

- RGB Fruit Kababs (Red, Green, Blue)
- coffee

Dinner - Chicken Stir-Fry

- 3 ounces chicken breast, in strips
- 1 t-spoon sesame oil
- 1 t-spoon minced garlic
- ½ t-spoon grated fresh ginger
- 1 cup broccoli florets
- 1 small carrot, peeled and sliced thinly green tea

Nutritional facts: Kcal - 756, carbs - 29g, protein - 55.8g, fat - 18g

11. Day 11

- Servings - 1
- Cooking Time - 40-50 min

Breakfast - Fruit Parfaits

- 1 cup mixed fresh fruit
- ¼ cup low-fat granola
- ½ cup fat-free vanilla yogurt
- 1 cup skim milk
- healthy tea

Lunch

- Pasta

Snack

- ¼ cup low-fat ranch dressing
- 1 red pepper, seeded and cut into strips

Dinner

- Vegetable
- Lasagna

Nutritional facts: Kcal - 966, carbs - 77g, protein - 51.4g, fat - 22g

12. Day 12

- Servings - 1
- Cooking Time - about 1 hour

Breakfast

- Fruit Salad and green tea

Lunch

- Salmon with rosemary

Snack

- 1 t-spoon almond butter
- 1 slice whole-grain toast
- ½ small banana, sliced

Dinner - Pork Fajitas

- ½ small onion, sliced thinly
- ½ red pepper, seeded and sliced thinly
- ¼ pound pork tenderloin, cut into strips tossed with Spice mix
- ½ yellow pepper, seeded and sliced thinly
- 1 medium tomato
- 2 whole-wheat flour tortillas, warmed in the microwave

- 1 cup shredded lettuce
- 1 large mango, peeled, pitted, and cut into chunks
- ¼ cup shredded low-fat cheddar cheese
- 1 cup sparkling water

Nutritional facts: Kcal - 1312, carbs - 82g, protein - 55.3g, fat - 25g

13. Day 13

- Servings - 1
- Cooking Time - about 1 hour

Breakfast

- 1 whole-wheat bagel
- 1 cup fresh-squeezed orange juice
- 1 small tomato sliced
- 2 t-spoons light cream cheese
- 1 cup cubed melon
- healthy tea

Lunch

- Vegetable with Mozzarella

Snack

- 1 apple
- 1-ounce low-fat cheese

Dinner - Oven Roasted Chicken Breast

- 4 ounces chicken breast, baked at 350 degrees F for 20 minutes
- Cracked black pepper
- 1 t-spoon unsalted butter

- Baked sweet potato

Nutritional facts: Kcal - 795, carbs - 43g, protein - 66.7g, fat - 22g

14. Day 14

- Servings - 1
- Cooking Time - 15-20 min

Breakfast

- Pumpkin

Lunch

- Vegetable and Mozzarella

Snack

- 1 apple
- 1-ounce low-fat cheese

Dinner

- Vegetable Lasagna
- green tea

Nutritional facts: Kcal - 684, carbs - 26g, protein - 60g, fat - 16g

15. Day 15

- Servings - 1
- Cooking Time - about 1 hour

Breakfast

- Fruit Salad

Lunch

- Simple Rosemary Salmon

Snack

- 3 cups air-popped unsalted popcorn

Dinner

- Vegetable
- Lasagna

Nutritional facts: Kcal - 738, carbs - 12g, protein - 72.8g, fat - 17g

16. Day 16

- Servings - 1
- Cooking Time - about 1 hour

Breakfast

- ½ cup slivered almonds
- 1 piece whole-grain toast
- 1 cup fresh mixed fruits of your choice, mixed with 1 cup fat-free, low-calorie yogurt
- 1 cup fat-free milk
- 1 t-spoon almond
- green tea

Lunch - Chicken Stuffed Red Pepper

- 1 large red pepper (baked until soft in at 350 degrees F)
- ½ cup brown rice, cooked
- 4 ounces shredded chicken breast
- 1 small tomato, seeded and diced
- 1 green onion, chopped
- ¼ teaspoon minced garlic

Snack

- Shrimp with Mango

Dinner - Oven Roasted Chicken Breast

- Cracked black pepper
- 4 ounces chicken breast and baked at 350 degrees F for 25 minutes
- Baked sweet potato
- 1 teaspoon unsalted butter

Nutritional facts: Kcal - 1476, carbs - 84g, protein - 77.4g, fat - 25g

17. Day 17

- Servings - 1
- Cooking Time - 30-40 min

Breakfast

- Easy Breakfast with vegetables

Lunch

- Pasta

Snack

- 1 red pepper, seeded and cut into strips
- ¼ cup low-fat ranch dressing

Dinner - Pecan-Crusted Baked Halibut

- 4 ounces halibut
- ½ cup quinoa with
- ½ cup chopped tomato
- 1 t-spoon crushed pecans ice water

Nutritional facts: Kcal - 782, carbs - 14g, protein - 55.4g, fat - 20g

18. Day 18

- Servings – 1 - Cooking Time - 30-40 min

Breakfast

- Fruit Filled French Toast

Lunch

- Lightning-Fast Chicken Stir-Fry

Snack

- 1 cup baby carrots
- 1-ounce light cheese

Dinner - Chicken Soft Taco

- 1 multigrain tortilla
- 4 ounces cooked chopped chicken
- ½ ripe avocado
- ½ cup black beans
- 1 cup unsweetened applesauce
- ½ cup shredded iceberg lettuce
- ½ small tomato
- 1 cup green tea

Nutritional facts: Kcal - 1087, carbs - 66g, protein - 77.8g, fat - 24g

19. Day 19

- Servings - 1
- Cooking Time - 40-50 min

Breakfast

- Light breakfast on a vegetable base

Lunch

- Fish (preferably Salmon) and healthy chips

Snack

- 4 graham crackers
- 1 cup vanilla fat-free, low-calorie yogurt

Dinner - Grilled Pork Tenderloin

- 4 ounces grilled pork tenderloin rubbed with nutmeg and cinnamon
- 1 t-spoon fat-free plain yogurt
- 1 small baked potato
- 1 t-spoon sliced green onions
- ½ cup halved cherry tomatoes
- ½ red pepper
- Mixed green salad
- ½ cup cucumber slices

- ½ cup shredded carrot
- 2 t-spoon balsamic vinaigrette

Nutritional facts: Kcal - 842, carbs - 76g, protein - 79.2g, fat - 19.3g

20. Day 20

- Servings – 1 - Cooking Time - 1 hour 30 min

Breakfast

- Grapefruit

Lunch - Pasta Salad

- 1 cup cooked whole-wheat or rice pasta
- ½ cup sliced mushrooms
- 1 small tomato, chopped
- ⅓ cup chopped red onion
- ½ yellow pepper, seeded and chopped
- 2 t-spoon low-fat, low-sodium feta cheese
- 1 cup fresh fruit juice

Snack

- Piece of turkey

Dinner

- Roast Chicken

Nutritional facts: Kcal - 774, carbs - 49g, protein - 49.6g, fat - 24g

21. Day 21

- Servings - 1
- Cooking Time - 1 hour 30 min

Breakfast

- 1 medium peach
- 1 small whole-wheat pita with 2 t-spoon sodium-free peanut butter
- 1 cup fat-free milk
- green tea

Lunch - Waldorf Chicken Salad

- 3 ounces cooked chopped chicken
- 3 stalks celery
- 1 small tart apple, cored and chopped
- ½ cup halved green grapes
- 3 t-spoons fat-free plain yogurt
- 1 t-spoon dried cranberries
- 1 cup green tea
- 1 cup cantaloupe cubes

Snack

- Popcorn

Dinner - Baked Salmon with Braised Spinach

- 2 bunches spinach, washed and tossed in 1 t-spoon water in a large skillet over medium heat until wilted and bright green
- 4 ounces salmon fillet drizzled with 1 t-spoon pure maple syrup topped with 1 t-spoon sesame seeds and baked at 450 degrees F for 10 minutes
- ½ green onion
- 1 cup fresh squeezed lemonade

Nutritional facts: Kcal - 710, carbs - 51g, protein - 64.2g, fat - 15g

More Interesting Recipes

Here in this chapter, we will see more meal ideas with concrete recipes you can try while your IF. Keep in mind that there are different ones, so you can decide when to try it and implement it in your diet plan. Let's some of them below:

1. BUTTER DROP BISCUITS

Nutritional facts: Kcal - 467, carbs - 69g, protein - 6g, fat - 19g

INGREDIENTS

- 6 tbsp unsalted butter
- ½ cups unbleached all-purpose flour
- ¼ cup cake flour
- 1 tbsp granulated sugar
- 2 tsp baking powder
- 1 tsp baking soda
- 1 tsp kosher salt
- ¼ cup cold shortening, cut into pieces
- 1 cup cold buttermilk, any fat content

YIELD

- Makes 6 biscuits

MIXING TIME

- 5 minutes

BAKING

- 475°F for about 12 minutes

DIRECTIONS

1. Position a rack in the middle of the oven and preheat to 475°F.
2. In a heavy, 9-in ovenproof frying pan, melt the butter over low heat.
3. Set aside.
4. Sift both flours, the sugar, baking powder, baking soda, and salt into a large bowl. Scatter the shortening over the top.
5. Using your thumb and fingertips, two table knives, or a pastry blender, work the shortening into the flour mixture until flour-coated pea-sized pieces form.
6. There will still be some loose flour.
7. Make a well in the center, pour the buttermilk into the well, and use a large spoon to mix the buttermilk into the dry ingredients to form a soft dough.
8. Using a ¼-cup capacity ice cream scoop or the large spoon, drop 6 rounded scoops of dough into the prepared pan, spacing them about ½ in apart (drop 5 biscuits in a circle around the edge of the pan and 1 biscuit in the middle).

9. Using the large spoon, carefully turn over each biscuit to coat both sides with butter.

10. Bake until the tops are golden, about 12 minutes.

11. Serve warm, directly from the pan. The biscuits can be baked up to 3 hours ahead and left in the pan, covered loosely with aluminum foil.

12. To serve, preheat the oven to 275°F and reheat the covered biscuits until warm, about 10 minutes.

2. Bottoms-Up Cinnamon-Caramel Pinwheels

Nutritional facts: Kcal - 415, carbs - 77g, protein - 4.6g, fat - 8g

INGREDIENTS:

- Glaze
- 4 tbsp unsalted butter
- 2 tbsp honey
- ½ cup packed light brown sugar

Biscuit Dough

- 1½ cups unbleached all-purpose flour
- ½ cup cake flour
- 1 tbsp granulated sugar
- 1 tsp baking powder
- ½ tsp baking soda
- ¾ ¾ tsp kosher salt
- 6 tbsp unsalted butter, melted
- 1 cup sour cream
- ¼ cup buttermilk, any fat content

- Topping
- ¼ cup granulated sugar
- 1 tsp ground cinnamon
- 1 tbsp unsalted butter, melted

YIELD

- Makes 9 rolls

MIXING TIME

- 15 minutes

BAKING

- 350°F for about 25 minutes

This is the fast version of a sticky bun. Spread a brown sugar glaze in the bottom of a pan, pat out soft biscuit dough, roll up the dough with cinnamon sugar, and bake it. Then feast on the fastest, stickiest, cinnamon-swirl buns around.

DIRECTIONS

1. Position a rack in the middle of the oven and preheat to 350°F.
2. Line a 9-in round pan or baking dish with 2-in-high sides with parchment paper.
3. Make the glaze. In a medium saucepan, combine the butter, honey, and brown sugar over

medium heat and cook, stirring often, until the butter and sugar melt and the glaze is smooth.

4. Pour the glaze into the prepared pan, tilting the pan to spread it evenly over the bottom. Set aside.

5. Make the biscuit dough.

6. Sift together both flours, the sugar, baking powder, baking soda, and salt into a medium bowl.

7. Put about half of the flour mixture into a large bowl.

8. Add the butter, sour cream, and buttermilk to the flour mixture in the large bowl and stir with a large spoon until blended.

9. Add the remaining flour mixture to the large bowl and stir until it is incorporated and a soft, ragged dough forms.

10. With floured hands, gather up the dough and put it on a lightly floured work surface. Knead the dough about 10 strokes: push down and away with the heel of your hand against the surface, then fold the dough in half toward you, and rotate it a quarter turn, flouring the surface as necessary to prevent sticking.

11. The dough is ready when it looks fairly smooth, feels very soft, and there is no loose flour.

12. Pat the dough into a rectangle about 12 by 7 in and in thick.

13. Make the topping. In a small bowl, stir together the sugar and cinnamon.

14. Using a pastry brush, spread the butter evenly over the dough, leaving a 1-in border uncovered on all sides.

15. Sprinkle the cinnamon sugar evenly over the butter.

16. Using a thin, metal spatula to help lift the dough, and starting from a long side, roll up the dough, jelly-roll style, pressing the seam to seal. If any dough sticks to the surface, use the spatula to spread the dough back onto the dough cylinder.

17. Pinch the ends to seal.

18. The role will be about 11 in long.

19. Using a sharp knife, cut the cylinder crosswise into 9 rolls, each about 1¼ in thick.

20. Place them, with a cut side up, in the prepared pan, arranging 7 rolls around the edge of the pan and 2 rolls in the middle.

21. Pinch together any edges that separate.

22. Bake until the tops feel firm and the edges just start to brown, about 25 minutes.

23. Let cool in the pan on a wire rack for 5 minutes.

24. Turn out onto a serving plate and peel away the parchment.

25. Serve warm.

26. The pinwheels can be baked 1 day ahead, unmolded as directed, covered, and left at room temperature.

27. To serve, preheat the oven to 275°F and reheat the pinwheels, sticky side up, until warm, about 15 minutes.

CHOICES

Sprinkle ⅓ cup raisins or dried cranberries over the cinnamon sugar

3. Red Cabbage-Apple Cauliflower Gnocchi

Nutritional facts: Kcal - 122, carbs - 30g, protein - 3g, fat - 0.5g

Tender cabbage and a vibrant applesauce-mustard pan sauce are perfect pair for low-carb cauliflower gnocchi. Add diced chicken-apple sausage for extra protein.

Ingredients: 4 servings

- 3 cups shredded red cabbage
- 2 tablespoons water, divided1 tablespoon olive oil
- 1 (12 ounce) bag frozen cauliflower gnocchi
- ½ cup unsweetened applesauce
- 1 tablespoon Dijon mustard
- Freshly ground pepper to taste

DIRECTIONS:

1. Place cabbage in a large microwave-safe bowl or baking dish.
2. Add 1 tablespoon water.

3. Cover tightly and microwave on High until softened, about 5 minutes.

4. Heat oil in a large skillet over medium-high heat.

5. Add gnocchi and cook, stirring frequently, until browned, about 5 minutes.

6. Add cabbage and the remaining 1 tablespoon water; cover and cook, stirring occasionally, until the water evaporates.

7. Stir in applesauce and mustard and heat through.

8. Season with pepper

4. Chicken-Spaghetti Squash Bake

Nutritional facts: Kcal - 425, carbs - 35g, protein - 35g, fat - 15g

In this version of a chicken-and-broccoli casserole, spaghetti squash takes on a creamy texture when baked with cream of mushroom soup.

Ingredients: 8 servings

- 1 medium spaghetti squash (about 3 lbs.)
- 4 cups broccoli florets1 tablespoon canola oil
- 1 (10 ounce) package sliced mushrooms
- 1 medium onion, finely chopped
- 2 cloves garlic, minced
- ½ teaspoon dried thyme
- ½ teaspoon ground pepper
- 1 (10 ounce) cans reduced-sodium condensed cream of mushroom soup, such as Campbell's 25%
- Less Sodium1½ pounds boneless, skinless chicken breasts, cut into bite-size pieces
- ½ cup shredded extra-sharp

- Cheddar cheese

DIRECTIONS:

Prep: 55 m

Ready In: 1 h 40 m

1. Preheat oven to 375°F.
2. Coat two 8-inch-square baking dishes with cooking spray.
3. Halve squash lengthwise and scoop out the seeds.
4. Place cut-side down in a microwave-safe dish; add 2 Tbsp. water.
5. Microwave, uncovered, on High until the flesh can be scraped with a fork but is still tender-crisp, 10 to 12 minutes.
6. Scrape the strands onto a plate; set aside.
7. Place broccoli in the same microwave-safe dish; add 1 Tbsp. water and cover.
8. Microwave on High, stirring occasionally, until just barely tender-crisp, 2 to 3 minutes.
9. Drain and set aside to cool.
10. Meanwhile, heat oil in a large nonstick skillet over medium-high heat.

11. Add mushrooms and cook, stirring, until they've released their juices, about 8 minutes.

12. Add onion and continue cooking until the onion is tender and the mushrooms are lightly browned, about 8 minutes.

13. Stir in garlic, thyme, and pepper; cook, stirring, for 30 seconds, Stir in soup (do not dilute with water) and heat through.

14. Stir in chicken and the reserved squash and broccoli, then gently toss to combine well.

15. Divide the mixture between the prepared baking dishes and sprinkle each with ¼ cup Cheddar.

16. Cover with foil.

17. Label and freeze one casserole for up to 1 month.

18. Bake the remaining casserole until bubbling, about 25 minutes.

19. Uncover and continue baking until lightly browned along the edges, 10 to 15 minutes more.

20. Let stand for 10 minutes before serving.

To make ahead: This double-batch recipe makes one casserole for tonight and one to freeze for up to 1 month (see Step 6). To cook from frozen: Thaw overnight in the refrigerator. Spoon off any liquid that has accumulated in the pan, if desired. Bake as directed in Step 7.

Equipment: Two 8-inch-square baking dishes or foil pans

5. Loaded Black Bean Nacho Soup

Nutritional facts: Kcal - 152, carbs - 27g, protein - 5.2g, fat - 2.2g

Jazz up a can of black bean soup with your favorite nacho toppings, such as cheese, avocado and fresh tomatoes. A bit of smoked paprika adds a bold flavor kick, but you can swap in any warm spices you prefer, such as cumin or chili powder. Look for a soup that contains no more than 450 mg sodium per serving.

Ingredients: 2 servings

- 1 (18 ounce) carton low-sodium black bean soup
- ¼ teaspoon smoked paprika
- ½ teaspoon lime juice
- ½ cup halved grape tomatoes
- ½ cup shredded cabbage or slaw mix
- 2 tablespoons crumbled cotija cheese or other Mexican-style shredded cheese
- ½ medium avocado, diced
- 2 ounces baked tortilla chips

DIRECTIONS:

1. Pour soup into a small saucepan and stir in paprika.
2. Heat according to package directions.
3. Stir in lime juice.
4. Divide the soup between 2 bowls and top with tomatoes, cabbage (or slaw), cheese and avocado.
5. Serve with tortilla chips.

6. Pesto Shrimp Pasta

Nutritional facts: Kcal - 236, carbs - 25g, protein - 4.7g, fat - 3g

Ingredients: 4 servings

- 1 cup dried orzo (6 ounces)
- 4 teaspoons packaged pesto sauce mix, such as Knorr brand, divided
- 2 tablespoons olive oil, divided
- 1 pound peeled and deveined fresh or frozen medium shrimp, thawed
- 1 medium zucchini, halved lengthwise and sliced
- ⅛ teaspoon coarse salt
- ⅛ teaspoon freshly cracked pepper
- 1 lemon, halved
- 1 ounce shaved Parmesan cheese

DIRECTIONS:

1. Prepare orzo pasta according to package directions.

2. Drain; reserving ¼ cup of the pasta cooking water.
3. Stir 1 teaspoon of the pesto mix into the reserved cooking water; set aside.
4. While pasta is boiling, combine 3 teaspoons of the pesto mix and 1 tablespoon of the olive oil in a large resealable plastic bag.
5. Seal and shake to combine.
6. Add shrimp to bag; seal and turn to coat.
7. Set aside.
8. Cook zucchini in a large skillet in the remaining 1 tablespoon hot oil over medium-high heat for 1 to 2 minutes, stirring often.
9. Add the pesto-marinated shrimp to the skillet and cook for 4 to 5 minutes or until shrimp is opaque.
10. Add the cooked pasta to the skillet with the zucchini and shrimp mixture.
11. Stir in the reserved pasta water until absorbed, scraping up any seasoning in the bottom of the pan.
12. Season with salt and pepper.
13. Squeeze the lemon halves over the pasta just before serving. Top with Parmesan and serve.

7. Honey Mustard Salmon & Mango Quinoa

Nutritional facts: Kcal - 315, carbs - 17g, protein - 20g, fat - 13.4g

In this 30-minute dinner recipe, grilled, honey mustard-coated salmon is served with a tasty grain salad made with quinoa, mango, jalapeño and almonds.

Ingredients: 2 servings

- 1 (8 ounce) fresh or frozen skinless salmon fillet
- 2 teaspoons honey
- 2 teaspoons spicy brown mustard
- 1 large clove garlic, minced
- ⅔ cup cooked quinoa, room temperature
- ½ cup chopped fresh or frozen mango, thawed if frozen
- 1 to 2 tablespoons seeded and finely chopped fresh jalapeño chile pepper
- 1 tablespoon sliced almonds, toasted
- 1 teaspoon olive oil

- ⅛ teaspoon salt
- Pinch ground black pepper
- 2 tablespoons chopped fresh cilantro

DIRECTIONS:

1. Thaw salmon, if frozen.
2. Rinse fish and pat dry with paper towels.
3. In a small bowl, stir together honey, mustard and garlic.
4. Brush both sides of salmon with honey mixture.
5. For a gas or charcoal grill, place salmon on grill rack directly over medium heat.
6. Cover and grill for 4 to 6 minutes per ½-inch thickness of fish until salmon begins to flake when tested with a fork, turning once.
7. Meanwhile, in a medium bowl, stir together quinoa, mango, jalapeño pepper, almonds, olive oil, salt and black pepper.
8. Top with fresh cilantro. Serve salmon with quinoa.

Tips: Because chile peppers contain volatile oils that can burn your skin and eyes, avoid direct contact with them as much as possible. When working with chile peppers, wear plastic or rubber gloves. If your bare hands do touch the peppers, wash your hands and nails well with soap and warm water.

To toast nuts, spread in a shallow baking pan lined with parchment paper. Bake in a 350°F oven for 5 to 10 minutes or until golden, shaking pan once or twice.

9. Pork Tenderloin with Apple-Onion Chutney

Nutritional facts: Kcal - 268, carbs - 17g, protein - 28.4g, fat - 14.4g

If you'd like the chutney in this pork tenderloin recipe to be both sweet and tart, opt for sweet apples like red or golden delicious and sweet onion.

Ingredients: 2 servings

- 1 (8 ounce) piece pork tenderloin
- ⅛ teaspoon dried thyme, crushed
- ⅛- ¼ teaspoon pepper
- ¾ cup thinly sliced onion
- 8 ounces apples, cored and sliced
- ¼ cup water
- 2 tablespoons cider vinegar
- 1 teaspoon honey
- ¼ teaspoon salt
- ⅛ teaspoon ground cumin (optional)
- Chopped fresh thyme (optional)

DIRECTIONS:

1. Trim fat from pork.

2. Cut the meat in half crosswise.

3. Place each piece, cut side down, between two pieces of plastic wrap.

4. Working from center to edges, pound lightly with the flat side of a meat mallet to ½-inch thickness.

5. Remove the plastic wrap.

6. Sprinkle the meat with dried thyme and pepper.

7. Lightly coat an unheated large skillet with cooking spray.

8. Add the pork.

9. Cook over medium-high heat for 6 to 9 minutes or until a thermometer inserted in the pork registers 145°F, turning once halfway through cooking.

10. Transfer the pork to a plate.

11. Cover and keep warm.

12. For chutney, cook onion in the same skillet about 4 minutes or until tender, stirring occasionally.

13. Stir in apple slices, the water, vinegar, honey, salt, and cumin (if desired).

14. Bring to boiling; reduce heat.

15. Simmer, uncovered, for 4 to 5 minutes or until the liquid is almost evaporated and the apples are tender, stirring occasionally.

16. Return the pork to the skillet and heat through.

17. Divide the pork and chutney between two plates. If desired, garnish with fresh thyme.

9. Easy Pea & Spinach Carbonara

Nutritional facts: Kcal - 574, carbs - 32g, protein - 6.5g, fat - 27g

Fresh pasta cooks up faster than dried, making it a must-have for fast weeknight dinners like this luscious yet healthy meal. Eggs are the base of the creamy sauce. They don't get fully cooked, so use pasteurized-in-the-shell eggs if you prefer.

Ingredients: 4 servings

- 1 ½ tablespoons extra-virgin olive oil
- ½ cup panko breadcrumbs, preferably whole-wheat
- 1 small clove garlic, minced
- 8 tablespoons grated Parmesan cheese, divided
- 3 tablespoons finely chopped fresh parsley
- 3 large egg yolks1 large egg
- ½ teaspoon ground pepper
- ¼ teaspoon salt
- 1 (9 ounce) package fresh tagliatelle or linguine
- 8 cups baby spinach

- 1 cup peas (fresh or frozen)

DIRECTIONS:

1. Put 10 cups of water in a large pot and bring to a boil over high heat.
2. Meanwhile, heat oil in a large skillet over medium-high heat.
3. Add breadcrumbs and garlic; cook, stirring frequently, until toasted, about 2 minutes.
4. Transfer to a small bowl and stir in 2 tablespoons Parmesan and parsley.
5. Set aside.
6. Whisk the remaining 6 tablespoons Parmesan, egg yolks, egg, pepper and salt in a medium bowl.
7. Cook pasta in the boiling water, stirring occasionally, for 1 minute.
8. Add spinach and peas and cook until the pasta is tender, about 1 minute more.
9. Reserve ¼ cup of the cooking water.
10. Drain and place in a large bowl.
11. Slowly whisk the reserved cooking water into the egg mixture.
12. Gradually add the mixture to the pasta, tossing with tongs to combine.

13. Serve topped with the reserved breadcrumb mixture.

10. Hearty Tomato Soup with Beans & Greens

Nutritional facts: Kcal - 45, carbs - 12g, protein - 2.5g, fat - 2.2g

Garlicky kale and creamy white beans elevate simple canned tomato soup into a 10-minute lunch or dinner that really satisfies. Use a soup with tomato pieces for a heartier texture. Look for a brand that's low- or reduced-sodium, with no more than 450 mg sodium per serving

Ingredients: 4 servings

- 2 (14 ounce) cans low-sodium hearty-style tomato soup
- 1 tablespoon olive oil
- 3 cups chopped kale
- 1 teaspoon minced garlic
- ⅛ teaspoon crushed red pepper (optional)
- 1 (14 ounce) can no-salt-added cannellini beans, rinsed
- ¼ cup grated Parmesan cheese

DIRECTIONS:

1. Heat soup in a medium saucepan according to package directions; simmer over low heat as you prepare kale.

2. Heat oil in a large skillet over medium heat.

3. Add kale and cook, stirring, until wilted, 1 to 2 minutes.

4. Stir in garlic and crushed red pepper (if using) and cook for 30 seconds.

5. Stir the greens and beans into the soup and simmer until the beans are heated through, 2 to 3 minutes.

6. Divide the soup among 4 bowls.

7. Serve topped with Parmesan.

11. Curried Chickpea Stew

Nutritional facts: Kcal - 590, carbs - 25g, protein - 19g, fat - 3g

Who says a meatless meal isn't filling? Packed with fiber-rich vegetables and chickpeas, this fragrant stew satisfies.

Ingredients: 8 servings

- 1 (10 ounce) bag prewashed spinach or other sturdy greens
- 1 ½ tablespoons canola oil1 large onion, chopped
- 1 (2 inch) piece fresh ginger, peeled and minced
- ½-1 small jalapeño pepper, seeded and finely chopped
- 3 cloves garlic, minced
- 1 tablespoon curry powder
- 3 medium carrots, peeled and thinly sliced
- ½ medium head cauliflower, broken into bite-size florets (3 cups)

- 2 (15 ounce) cans low sodium chickpeas, rinsed
- 2 (14 ounce) cans no-salt-added diced tomatoes, drained
- ½ cup fat-free half-and-half
- ⅓ cup "lite" coconut milk

DIRECTIONS:

1. Place spinach (or other greens) in a microwave-safe dish; add 1 Tbsp. water and cover.
2. Microwave on High, stirring occasionally, until just wilted, 1 to 2 minutes.
3. Transfer to a colander to drain.
4. When cool enough to handle, squeeze out any excess water.
5. Coarsely chop and set aside. Heat oil in a large nonstick skillet with high sides or a Dutch oven.
6. Add onion and cook, stirring, until translucent, about 8 minutes.
7. Add ginger, jalapeño, garlic, and curry powder; cook, stirring, for 30 seconds.
8. Add carrots and 2 Tbsp. water; cover and cook, stirring occasionally, until the carrots have softened, about 10 minutes (add more water if the mixture becomes dry).

9. Add cauliflower; cover and cook, stirring occasionally, until barely tender-crisp, 5 to 10 minutes more.
10. Stir in chickpeas, tomatoes, half-and-half, and coconut milk.
11. Bring to just below boiling.
12. Reduce heat to low and simmer uncovered, stirring occasionally, for 15 minutes.
13. Stir in the reserved spinach (or greens) and heat through.
14. Transfer half of the mixture (about 5 cups) to a 1½-qt. freezer container; label and freeze for up to 1 month.
15. Serve the remaining half at once or refrigerate for up to 3 days.

To make ahead: This double-batch recipe makes one meal for tonight (or to refrigerate for up to 3 days) and one to freeze for up to 1 month (see Step 4).

To cook from frozen: Thaw overnight in the refrigerator, then microwave on High until heated through, 4 to 5 minutes. You can also reheat the stew in a saucepan until bubbling; add a little water, if needed, to prevent sticking.

12. Pork & Green Chile Stew

Nutritional facts: Kcal - 270, carbs - 2.7g, protein - 1.5g, fat - 2.3g

Let your slow cooker work—while you're at work!—and come home to a delicious bowl of hearty stew for dinner. Full of potatoes, hominy, green chiles, and chunks of pork sirloin, this filling stew recipe takes just 25 minutes to prepare in the morning.

Ingredients: 6 servings

- 2 pounds boneless pork sirloin roast or shoulder roast
- 1 tablespoon vegetable oil
- ½ cup chopped onion (1 medium)
- 4 cups peeled and cubed potatoes (4 medium)
- 3 cups water
- 1 (15 ounce) can hominy or whole kernel corn, drained
- 2 (4 ounce) cans diced green chile peppers, undrained
- 2 tablespoons quick-cooking tapioca

- 1 teaspoon garlic salt
- ½ teaspoon ground cumin
- ½ teaspoon ancho chile powder
- ½ teaspoon ground pepper
- ¼ teaspoon dried oregano, crushed
- Chopped fresh cilantro (optional)

DIRECTIONS:

1. Trim fat from meat.
2. Cut the meat into ½-inch pieces.
3. Cook half of the meat in a large skillet in hot oil over medium-high heat until browned.
4. Using a slotted spoon, remove the meat from the skillet.
5. Repeat with the remaining meat and the onion.
6. Drain off fat.
7. Transfer all of the meat and the onion to a 3½- to 4½-quart slow cooker.
8. Stir in potatoes, the water, hominy, green chile peppers, tapioca, garlic salt, cumin, ancho chile powder, ground pepper, and oregano.
9. Cover and cook on Low for 7 to 8 hours or on High for 4 to 5 hours. If desired, garnish each serving with cilantro.

10. **Equipment**: 3½- to 4½-quart slow cooker

13. Trapanese Pesto Pasta & Zoodles with Salmon

Nutritional facts: Kcal - 643, carbs - 25g, protein - 25g, fat - 14.2g

Trapanese pesto is the Sicilian version of the sauce that uses tomatoes and almonds instead of pine nuts. This savory pesto sauce coats low-carb zucchini noodles and heart-healthy seared salmon to create an absolutely delicious pasta dinner.

Ingredients: 6 servings

- 2 zucchini (1¾ lbs. total)
- 1 teaspoon salt, divided
- ½ cup raw whole almonds, toasted
- 1 pound grape tomatoes (3 cups)
- 1 cup packed fresh basil leaves plus ¼ cup chopped, divided
- 2-4 cloves garlic¼ teaspoon crushed red pepper
- 3 tablespoons olive oil, divided
- 8 ounces whole-wheat spaghetti

- 1 pound skinless salmon fillets (about 4 fillets), patted dry
- ¼ teaspoon ground pepper, plus more for garnish
- 2 tablespoons grated Parmesan cheese (optional)

Preparation:

1. Bring a large pot of water to a boil.
2. Cut zucchini into long thin strips with a spiralizer or vegetable peeler.
3. Place in a colander set over a large bowl.
4. Toss with ¼ tsp. salt and let drain for 15 to 20 minutes.
5. Meanwhile, pulse almonds in a food processor until coarsely chopped.
6. Add tomatoes, 1 cup basil leaves, garlic, and crushed red pepper; pulse until coarsely chopped.
7. Add 2 Tbsp. oil and ½ tsp. salt and pulse until combined; set aside.
8. Cook spaghetti in the boiling water according to package directions.
9. Drain and transfer to a large bowl.

10. Gently squeeze the zucchini to remove excess water; add to the bowl with the spaghetti.

11. Heat the remaining 1 Tbsp. oil in a large skillet over medium-high heat until shimmering.

12. Season salmon with pepper and the remaining ¼ tsp. salt.

13. Add the salmon to the pan; cook until the underside is golden and crispy, about 4 minutes.

14. Flip the salmon and cook until it flakes when nudged with a fork, 2 to 4 minutes more.

15. Transfer to a plate and use a fork to gently flake it apart.

16. Add the pesto to the spaghetti mixture; toss to coat.

17. Gently stir in the salmon.

18. Top with the remaining ¼ cup chopped fresh basil.

19. Garnish with Parmesan and additional pepper, if desired.

14. Chicken & Pineapple Slaw

Nutritional facts: Kcal - 285, carbs - 15g, protein - 27.5g, fat - 14.8g

Ready in under 30 minutes, this spicy chicken dish with sweet pinapple slaw is perfect for any night of the week.

Ingredients: 4 servings

- 3 heads baby bok choy, trimmed and thinly sliced
- 2 cups shredded red cabbage
- ½ of a fresh pineapple, peeled, cored and chopped
- 2 tablespoons cider vinegar
- 4 teaspoons packed brown sugar
- 2 teaspoons all-purpose flour
- 2 teaspoons jerk seasoning
- 4 skinless, boneless chicken breast halves (1 to 1¼ pounds total)

DIRECTIONS:

1. For pineapple slaw, in a very large bowl combine bok choy, cabbage and pineapple.
2. In a small bowl combine cider vinegar and 2 teaspoons of the brown sugar.
3. Drizzle over bok choy mixture; toss to coat.
4. Set aside.
5. In a large resealable plastic bag combine the remaining 2 teaspoons brown sugar, the flour and jerk seasoning.
6. Add chicken; shake well to coat.
7. Grease a grill pan or a heavy 12-inch skillet.
8. Add chicken; cook over medium heat for 8 to 12 minutes or until no longer pink (170°F), turning once halfway through cooking time.
9. Transfer chicken to a cutting board.
10. Slice chicken and serve with pineapple slaw.

15. Jambalaya Stuffed Peppers

Nutritional facts: Kcal - 376, carbs - 52g, protein - 16g, fat - 12g

In this healthy stuffed peppers recipe, a delicious jambalaya filling of chicken and Cajun spices gets baked inside of bell peppers. Traditional jambalaya is made with green bell peppers, but you can use green, yellow, or orange peppers (or a mix) for this dish. Look for bell peppers with even bottoms, so that they stand upright on their own.

Ingredients: 6 servings

- 6 large green, yellow, or orange bell peppers
- 1½ pounds boneless, skinless chicken thighs, trimmed and cut into 1-inch pieces
- 2 tablespoons salt-free Cajun seasoning, divided
- 2 tablespoons olive oil, divided
- 1 link andouille sausage (3-4 oz.), sliced
- ½ cup diced celery1 small onion, diced (½ cup)
- 2 cloves garlic, minced½ teaspoon salt
- 1 (14 ounce) can diced tomatoes

- ¼ cup tomato paste1 cup low-sodium chicken broth
- 1 cup uncooked instant brown rice

DIRECTIONS:

1. Preheat oven to 400°F.
2. Line a large rimmed baking sheet with parchment paper or foil.
3. Cut tops off peppers and carefully remove the core and seeds, taking care not to split the skin.
4. Dice the pepper tops and set aside.
5. Place the peppers on the prepared baking sheet; bake for 20 minutes.
6. Remove from oven and let cool.
7. Discard any accumulated liquid in the bottom of the peppers.
8. Meanwhile, season chicken on all sides with 1 Tbsp. Cajun seasoning.
9. Heat 1 Tbsp. oil on a large skillet over medium heat.
10. Add half of the chicken and cook, turning to brown all sides, 4 to 6 minutes.
11. Transfer the chicken to a medium bowl with a slotted spoon.

12. Repeat with the remaining 1 Tbsp. olive oil and the remaining chicken.

13. Add sausage to the now-empty skillet and cook, stirring occasionally, until lightly browned, 1 to 2 minutes.

14. Add celery, onion, and the reserved diced pepper; cook, stirring often, until the onions are translucent, 3 to 5 minutes.

15. Add garlic, the remaining 1 Tbsp. Cajun seasoning, and salt; cook, stirring, for 30 seconds.

16. Add tomatoes and tomato paste; stir to combine, scraping any brown bits off the bottom of the pan.

17. Add broth, rice, and the chicken with any accumulated juices; stir to combine.

18. Bring to a boil.

19. Reduce heat to maintain a simmer and cook, stirring occasionally, until the chicken has cooked through and the rice has softened, 5 to 10 minutes.

20. Remove from heat and stir.

21. Let stand, covered, until all liquid is absorbed, about 10 minutes.

22. Divide the chicken mixture among the peppers, spooning about 1¼ cups into each one and mounding it on top, if necessary.

23. Bake until heated through, about 20 minutes.

Tip: Homemade Cajun seasoning is recommended, because it has more flavor and fewer preservatives than the store-bought versions. For salt-free Cajun seasoning, mix 1 Tbsp. paprika, 1 tsp. each onion powder and garlic powder, ½ tsp. each dried oregano and thyme, and ¼ tsp. each cayenne and ground pepper. You will have slightly more than you need for this recipe; use it to season eggs, chicken, fish, or vegetables. (Want to have extra on hand? Multiply these amounts by four.) Store in a covered jar for up to 6 months.

16. Spinach, Apple & Chicken Salad with Poppy Seed Dressing & Cheese Crisps

---

Nutritional facts: Kcal - 684, carbs - 74g, protein - 27.5g, fat - 18.8g

Ingredients 4 servings

- 3 9-by-14-inch phyllo pastry sheets, thawed
- 4 teaspoons extra-virgin olive oil plus 2 tablespoons, divided
- 1 large egg white, beaten
- ⅓ cup freshly grated Parmigiano-Reggiano cheese
- 1 tablespoon fresh thyme leaves
- 3 tablespoons buttermilk
- 2 tablespoons honey
- 1 tablespoon cider vinegar
- 1 teaspoon poppy seeds
- ½ teaspoon Dijon mustard
- ½ teaspoon kosher salt
- 5 cups baby spinach

- 1 ½ cups shredded cooked chicken breast
- 1 medium Gala apple, sliced

DIRECTIONS:

1. Preheat oven to 350°F.
2. Line a baking sheet with parchment paper.
3. Place 1 sheet of phyllo on the prepared baking sheet.
4. Brush with 2 teaspoons oil.
5. Top with a second sheet of phyllo, pressing gently to adhere.
6. Brush with 2 teaspoons oil.
7. Place the third sheet on top and brush with egg white.
8. Sprinkle with cheese and thyme.
9. Using a pizza cutter or sharp knife, cut the phyllo stack into approximately 2-inch squares.
10. Bake until golden brown, about 8 minutes.
11. Let cool for about 3 minutes.
12. Meanwhile, whisk the remaining 2 tablespoons oil, buttermilk, honey, vinegar, poppy seeds, mustard and salt in a medium bowl.
13. Add spinach, chicken and apple to the bowl and toss to coat.
14. Serve with the phyllo crisps.

To make ahead: Refrigerate dressing (Step 3) for up to 2 days. **Equipment**: Parchment paper

17. Hazelnut-Parsley Roast Tilapia

Nutritional facts: Kcal - 856, carbs - 20g, protein - 16.7g, fat - 68g

Sweet and crunchy hazelnuts team up with bright lemon and fresh parsley to add oomph to the tilapia for an easy seafood recipe. Serve this atop a salad or alongside brown rice or orzo.

Ingredients: 4 servings

- 2 tablespoons olive oil, divided
- 4 (5 ounce) tilapia fillets (fresh or frozen, thawed
- ⅓ cup finely chopped hazelnuts
- ¼ cup finely chopped fresh parsley
- 1 small shallot, minced
- 2 teaspoons lemon zest
- ⅛ teaspoon salt plus ¼ teaspoon, divided
- ¼ teaspoon ground pepper, divided
- 1½ tablespoons lemon juice

DIRECTIONS:

1. Preheat oven to 450°F.
2. Line a large rimmed baking sheet with foil; brush with 1 Tbsp. oil.
3. Bring fish to room temperature by letting it stand on the counter for 15 minutes.
4. Meanwhile, stir together hazelnuts, parsley, shallot, lemon zest, 1 tsp. oil, ⅛ tsp. salt, and ⅛ tsp. pepper in a small bowl.
5. Pat both sides of the fish dry with a paper towel.
6. Place the fish on the prepared baking sheet. Brush both sides of the fish with lemon juice and the remaining 2 tsp. oil.
7. Season both sides evenly with the remaining ¼ tsp. salt and ⅛ tsp. pepper.
8. Divide the hazelnut mixture evenly among the tops of the fillets and pat gently to adhere.
9. Roast the fish until it is opaque, firm, and just beginning to flake, 7 to 10 minutes.
10. Serve immediately.

18. Charred Vegetable & Bean Tostadas

Nutritional facts: Kcal - 457, carbs - 77g, protein - 25g, fat - 2.6g

Pile vegetables and black beans onto crisp tostadas and top them off with lime crema for a vegetarian dinner the whole family will love. Charring the vegetables under the broiler infuses them with smoky flavor while cooking them quickly.

Ingredients: 6 servings

- Lime Crema
- 5 tablespoons sour cream
- ⅛ teaspoon lime zest
- 2teaspoons lime juice
- ⅛ teaspoon kosher salt
- Tostadas
- 6corn tortillas
- 2tablespoons canola oil plus 2 teaspoons, divided

- 4cloves garlic, sliced, divided
- 1½ teaspoons ground cumin
- 1teaspoon kosher salt, divided
- ⅛ teaspoon chipotle chile powder
- 2(15 ounce) cans no-salt-added black beans, rinsed
- ¼ cup water, plus more as needed
- 2medium red bell peppers, sliced
- 1large red onion, halved and sliced
- 2medium zucchini, halved and sliced
- ½ inch thick
- 1cup fresh or frozen corn kernels
- ¼ teaspoon ground pepper
- 1 cup thinly shredded cabbage
- ¼ cup chopped fresh cilantro
- 6 tablespoons crumbled cotija cheese

DIRECTIONS:

To prepare crema: Combine sour cream, lime zest, lime juice and salt in a small bowl. Set aside.

To prepare tostadas:

1. Position a rack in upper third of oven; preheat to 400°F.

2. Brush both sides of tortillas with 1 tablespoon oil and arrange on a baking sheet. (It's OK if they overlap a bit; they will shrink as they cook.)

3. Bake, turning once halfway, until browned and crisp, about 10 minutes.

4. Transfer to a wire rack and let cool. Meanwhile, heat 2 teaspoons oil in a large skillet over medium heat.

5. Add 1 garlic clove and cook, stirring occasionally, until fragrant, about 30 seconds.

6. Add cumin, ½ teaspoon salt and chile powder; cook, stirring, for 30 seconds more.

7. Add beans and cook, stirring occasionally, until heated through, about 4 minutes.

8. Transfer the beans to a food processor and add ¼ cup water.

9. Pulse until smooth, adding more water, 1 tablespoon at a time, if needed.

10. Preheat broiler to high.

11. Toss bell peppers, onion, zucchini, corn, ground pepper, the remaining 3 garlic cloves, 1 tablespoon oil and ½ teaspoon salt in a large bowl.

12. Spread on a large rimmed baking sheet.

13. Broil, stirring occasionally, until lightly charred, 8 to 12 minutes.
14. Top the tostadas with some of the beans, charred vegetables, cabbage, cilantro, cheese and the reserved crema.

19. Pistachio-Crusted Baked Trout

Nutritional facts: Kcal - 155, carbs - 10g, protein - 25g, fat - 7.5g

Finely chopped pistachios take center stage in this baked fish recipe. The toasted seeds are mixed to create fragrant and crunchy crust which nicely includes the tender fish.

Ingredients: 4 servings

- 4 (4-5 ounce) fresh or frozen trout fillets
- ½ teaspoon coriander seeds
- ½ teaspoon cumin seeds
- ½ teaspoon caraway seeds
- 4 teaspoons olive oil
- 1 teaspoon finely shredded lemon peel
- 1 clove garlic, minced
- ½ teaspoon kosher salt
- ¼ teaspoon ground cinnamon
- ¼ teaspoon ground pepper
- ¼ cup pistachio nuts, finely chopped
- 4 lemon wedges

DIRECTIONS:

1. Thaw fish, if frozen.
2. Preheat oven to 350°F.
3. Line a shallow baking pan with foil and coat with cooking spray; set aside.
4. Heat a small saucepan over low heat; add coriander seeds, cumin seeds, and caraway seeds.
5. Cook and stir for 4 minutes or until fragrant and golden. (Do not allow the seeds to burn or they will taste bitter.)
6. Remove from heat.
7. Using a small food processor or a mortar and pestle, grind the seeds.
8. Stir in oil, lemon peel, garlic, salt, cinnamon, and pepper.
9. Place pistachios in a small bowl; set aside.
10. Rinse the fish; pat dry with paper towels.
11. Spread one side of the fish fillets with the spice mixture.
12. Bringing up two opposite ends, fold the fish into thirds.

13. Dip the top and the sides of the fish bundles into the nuts to coat; place in the prepared baking pan.
14. Sprinkle with any remaining nuts.
15. Bake for 15 to 20 minutes or until the fish begins to flake when tested with a fork (145°F).
16. Serve with lemon wedges.

Tip: Save some time by asking your butcher or fishmonger to fillet the fish and remove the skin.

20. Pork Medallions with Cranberry-Onion Relish

Nutritional facts: Kcal - 157, carbs - 7g, protein - 32g, fat - 3.5g

Pork tenderloin is a great choice for dinner when it's thinly sliced into quick-cooking medallions. A tart cranberry and onion relish adds delicious taste to each bite of this 30-minute entree.

Ingredients: 4 servings

- 12 ounces pork tenderloin
- ¼ cup all-purpose flour
- Pinch of salt
- Pinch of ground pepper
- 2 tablespoons olive oil, divided
- 1 small onion, thinly sliced
- ¼ cup dried cranberries
- ¼ cup reduced-sodium chicken broth
- 1 tablespoon balsamic vinegar

DIRECTIONS:

1. Trim fat from pork.
2. Cut the pork crosswise into eight slices.
3. Place each slice between two pieces of plastic wrap.
4. Using the flat side of a meat mallet, lightly pound the pork to ¼-inch thickness.
5. Discard plastic wrap.
6. Combine flour, salt, and pepper in a shallow dish.
7. Dip the pork slices into the flour mixture, turning to coat.
8. Coat a heavy large skillet with cooking spray.
9. Add 1 tablespoon oil to the skillet; heat over medium-high heat.
10. Add four pork slices to the hot oil; cook for 3 to 4 minutes or until the pork is slightly pink in the center, turning once halfway through the cooking time.
11. Transfer the pork to a serving platter; cover with foil to keep warm.
12. Repeat with the remaining 1 tablespoon oil and the remaining four pork slices.

13. Cook onion in the same skillet over medium heat for about 4 minutes or until crisp-tender.
14. Combine cranberries, broth, and vinegar in a small bowl; carefully add to the skillet.
15. Heat through.
16. Serve the onion mixture over the pork slices.

21. Lemon Chicken & Rice

Nutritional facts: Kcal - 370, carbs - 28g, protein - 29.2g, fat - 14.5g

This easy persian-inspired chicken and rice dish has a beautiful golden color and a wonderful fragrance. If you have saffron in the cupboard, do add that optional pinch; just a little will enhance the flavor and aroma of the dish.

Ingredients: 8 servings

- 2 tablespoons olive oil, divided
- 8 boneless, skinless chicken thighs (1¼-1½ lbs. total), trimmed
- 2 large onions, thinly sliced
- ½ teaspoon salt, divided3 cloves garlic, minced
- 2 teaspoons ground turmeric
- 1 teaspoon paprika
- Generous pinch of saffron (optional)
- 3 cups shredded cabbage (about ½ small head)
- 4 cups cooked brown rice, preferably basmati or jasmine

- ¼ cup lemon juice
- 2 tablespoons chopped fresh Italian parsley (optional)
- 1 lemon, sliced (optional)

DIRECTIONS:

Prep: 50 m

Ready In: 1 h 35 m

1. Preheat oven to 375°F.
2. Coat two 8-inch-square baking dishes or foil pans with cooking spray.
3. Heat 1 Tbsp. oil in a large nonstick skillet over medium-high heat.
4. Add 4 chicken thighs, and cook, turning once, until both sides are lightly browned, about 4 minutes.
5. Transfer the chicken to a plate and set aside.
6. Repeat with the remaining chicken thighs.
7. Pour off all but about 1 Tbsp. fat from the pan.
8. Add the remaining 1 Tbsp. oil and onions to the pan and sprinkle with ¼ tsp. salt.
9. Cook, stirring, until soft and golden, 12 to 15 minutes.

10. Stir in garlic, turmeric, paprika, and saffron, if using; cook, stirring, for 2 minutes.

11. Transfer the onions to a plate and set aside.

12. Return the pan to medium-high heat and add cabbage.

13. Cook, stirring, until wilted, about 3 minutes.

14. Stir in rice, lemon juice, the remaining ¼ tsp. salt, and half of the reserved onion.

15. Continue cooking until the rice is well coated and heated through, 5 to 7 minutes.

16. Divide the rice mixture between the prepared baking dishes; nestle 4 of the reserved chicken thighs in each dish.

17. Top each with half of the remaining cooked onions.

18. Cover both dishes with foil.

19. Label one and freeze for up to 1 month.

20. Bake the remaining casserole, covered, for 30 minutes.

21. Uncover and continue baking until a thermometer inserted in the thickest part of the chicken registers 165°F and the onions are starting to brown around the edges, 5 to 10 minutes more.

22. Garnish with parsley and lemon slices, if desired.

Tip: Instead of freezing half, you can bake the full recipe in a 9x13-inch baking pan. In Step 6, bake, covered, for an additional 10 minutes.

To make ahead: This double-batch recipe makes one meal for tonight and one to freeze for up to 1 month (see Step 5). To cook from frozen: Thaw overnight in the refrigerator, then bake as directed in Steps 6-7, adding an additional 10 minutes baking time once uncovered.

Equipment: Two 8-inch-square baking dishes or foil pans

22. Toasted Pecan & Chocolate Chunk Scones

Nutritional facts: Kcal - 1250, carbs - 74g, protein - 32g, fat - 86g

INGREDIENTS:

- 2 cups unbleached all-purpose flour
- ¼ cup granulated sugar
- 1¼ tsp baking powder
- ¼ tsp baking soda
- ¼ tsp kosher salt
- ½ cup cold unsalted butter, cut into 16 pieces
- cup buttermilk, any fat content
- 2 tbsp pure maple syrup
- 3 oz semisweet chocolate, chopped
- ½ cup pecans, toasted and coarsely chopped
- 1 large egg lightly beaten with 1 tbsp heavy cream for egg wash
- Vanilla whipped cream for serving (optional)

YIELD

- Makes 8 scones

MIXING TIME

- 10 minutes

BAKING

- 400°F for about 18 minutes

DIRECTIONS:

1. Position a rack in the middle of the oven and preheat to 400°F.
2. Line a baking sheet with parchment paper.
3. In a large bowl, whisk together the flour, sugar, baking powder, baking soda, and salt. Scatter the butter pieces over the top.
4. Using your thumb and fingertips, two table knives, or a pastry blender, work the butter into the flour mixture until flour-coated pea-sized pieces form. There will still be some loose flour.
5. Make a well in the center, pour the buttermilk and maple syrup into the well, and use a large spoon to mix them into the dry ingredients to form a soft dough.
6. Stir in the chocolate and pecans.

7. With floured hands, gather up the dough and put it on a lightly floured work surface. Knead the dough about 5 strokes: push down and away with the heel of your hand against the surface, then fold the dough in half toward you, and rotate it a quarter turn, flouring the surface as necessary to prevent sticking.

8. The dough is ready when it looks smooth, feels soft, and there is no loose flour.

9. Lightly flour the work surface again and pat the dough into a 7-in circle 1¼ in thick.

10. Cut the circle into 8 wedges by cutting it into quarters and then cutting the quarters in half.

11. Use a wide spatula to transfer the scones to the prepared baking sheet, spacing them about 1½ in apart.

12. Using a pastry brush, brush the tops with the egg wash. (You will not use all of the eggwash). Bake until the tops are lightly browned and the bottoms are browned, about 18 minutes.

13. Transfer to a wire rack to cool for at least 15 minutes before serving.

14. Accompany with whipped cream, if desired.

15. The scones can be baked 1 day ahead, covered, and stored at room temperature.
16. To serve, preheat the oven to 275°F and reheat the scones until warm, about 15 minutes.

22. Chetty & Almond Whole-Wheat Scones

Nutritional facts: Kcal - 220, carbs - 15g, protein - 7g, fat - 14.3g

INGREDIENTS

- 1½ cups unbleached all-purpose flour
- ½ cup whole-wheat flour
- ½ cup granulated sugar, plus 2 tsp
- 1 tsp baking powder
- 1 tsp baking soda
- ½ tsp kosher salt
- 1 tsp ground cinnamon
- 1 tsp grated orange zest
- ½ cup cold unsalted butter, cut into 16 pieces
- 1 tsp pure vanilla extract
- ½ tsp pure almond extract
- ¾ cup buttermilk, any fat content
- ½ cup dried pitted cherries
- 1 large egg, lightly beaten, for egg wash

- 3 tbsp natural or blanched sliced almonds or coarsely chopped natural
- almonds
- Cherry jam and butter or clotted cream for serving

YIELD

- Makes 8 scones

MIXING TIME

- 10 minutes

BAKING

- 400°F for about 15 minutes

A bit of whole-wheat flour for flavor and fiber, always-in-season dried cherries, and a sweet crunchy almond topping makes these scones worth trying. Although the outside bakes up crisp, the dough is quite soft and can be patted out rather than rolled. A soft dough makes the inside of the scone especially moist and tender. These scones will spread quite a bit during baking, so be sure to give them adequate space on the pan.

DIRECTIONS:

1. Position a rack in the middle of the oven and preheat to 400°F.

2. Line a baking sheet with parchment paper.

3. In a large bowl, whisk together both flours, the ½ cup sugar, the baking powder, baking soda, salt, and cinnamon.

4. Stir in the orange zest.

5. Scatter the butter pieces over the top.

6. Using your thumb and fingertips, two table knives, or a pastry blender, work the butter into the flour mixture until flour-coated pea-sized pieces form.

7. There will still be some loose flour.

8. Make a well in the center, add the buttermilk, vanilla, almond extract, and cherries to the well, and use a large spoon to mix them into the dry ingredients to form a soft dough.

9. With floured hands, gather the dough into a softball, put it on a floured rolling surface, and pat into an 8-in circle about ¾ in thick.

10. Cut the circle into 8 wedges by cutting it into quarters and then cutting the quarters in half.

11. Use a wide spatula to transfer the scones to the prepared baking sheet, placing them about 3 in apart.

12. Using a pastry brush, brush the tops with the egg wash. (You will not use all of the egg wash).

13. Sprinkle the almonds evenly over the top, pressing them gently onto the dough.

14. Sprinkle the remaining 2 tsp sugar over the nuts.

15. Bake until the tops are lightly colored, the edges are lightly browned, and the bottoms are browned about 15 minutes.

16. Transfer to a wire rack to cool for at least 15 minutes before serving.

17. Accompany with jam and butter.

18. The scones can be baked 1 day ahead, covered, and left at room temperature.

19. To serve, preheat the oven to 275°F and reheat the scones until warm, about 15 minutes.

23. Pumpkin-Chocolate Chip Pancakes

Nutritional facts: Kcal - 56, carbs - 13g, protein - 18g, fat - 5g

INGREDIENTS

- 1 cup unbleached all-purpose flour
- 1 tsp baking powder
- ½ tsp baking soda
- ¼ tsp kosher salt
- 1 tsp ground cinnamon
- ½ tsp ground ginger
- ¾ cup milk, any fat content
- 1 large egg
- 3 tbsp pure maple syrup
- ¾ cup canned pumpkin
- ¼ cup full-fat or low-fat plain yogurt
- cup semisweet chocolate chips, or 4 ½ oz semisweet chocolate, chopped
- 2 tbsp unsalted butter

- 1 cup vanilla yogurt for serving

YIELD

- Makes twelve 4-in pancakes

MIXING TIME

- 10 minutes

COOKING

- 4½ to 6 minutes per batch

I have never understood pancake mixes. Homemade pancake batter is fast and easy to mix and allows so many interesting variations. These pancakes, which are a rich pumpkin color, are sweetened with maple syrup, spiced with cinnamon and ginger, and include warm chocolate chips in every bite.

DIRECTIONS:

1. Sift together the flour, baking powder, baking soda, salt, cinnamon, and ginger into a medium bowl.
2. Make a well in the center and add the milk, egg, maple syrup, pumpkin, and plain yogurt to the well.

3. Using a large spoon, stir the batter just until all the ingredients are blended and there is no loose flour.

4. You may see some small lumps; that's okay.

5. Stir in the chocolate chips just until evenly distributed.

6. Preheat the oven to 250° F.

7. You will be keeping the first batches of pancakes warm in the oven until all the batter is used.

8. Heat a griddle or large frying pan over medium heat, and add 1 tbsp of the butter.

9. Using a pastry brush (preferably silicone), spread the butter evenly over the surface. Using 3 tbsp for each pancake, ladle the batter onto the hot griddle, being careful not to crowd the pancakes.

10. After 3 to 4 minutes, when bubbles

11. have formed near the edges of the pancakes (they will not bubble in the center), the edges have begun to look dry, and the underside is golden brown, carefully turn the pancakes with a spatula.

12. Cook until lightly browned on the second sides, 1½ to 2 minutes longer.

13. Transfer to an ovenproof platter in a single layer and place in the oven.

14. Do not cover the pancakes or they will become get soggy.

15. Repeat with the remaining batter, adding additional butter to the griddle as needed.

16. Serve the pancakes hot and pass the vanilla yogurt at the table for 2 to 4 people.

24. Pumpkin Seed Salmon with Maple-Spice

Nutritional facts: Kcal - 654, carbs - 55g, protein - 39, fat - 32g

Because this one-pan meal is ready in just 35 minutes, it's a good choice for a healthy recipe after you've had a long day at the office. Maple-spiced carrots cook alongside pepita-crusted salmon fillets and deliver amazing taste and nutrition in a dinner the whole family will devour.

Ingredients: 4 servings

- 4 (4-5 ounce) fresh or frozen salmon fillets
- 1-pound carrots, cut diagonally into ¼-inch slices
- ¼ cup pure maple syrup, divided½ teaspoon salt, divided
- ½ teaspoon pumpkin pie spice
- 8 multi-grain saltine crackers, finely crushed

- 3 tablespoons finely chopped salted, roasted pumpkin seeds (pepitas) plus 2 teaspoons, divided
- Cooking spray

DIRECTIONS:

1. Thaw fish, if frozen.
2. Preheat oven to 425°F.
3. Line a 15x10-inch baking pan with foil; set aside.
4. Combine carrots, 3 tablespoons maple syrup, ¼ teaspoon salt, and the pumpkin pie spice in a large bowl.
5. Arrange the carrots on one-half of the prepared baking pan.
6. Bake for 10 minutes.
7. Meanwhile, rinse the fish; pat dry with paper towels.
8. Combine crushed crackers, 3 tablespoons of the pumpkin seeds, and the remaining ¼ teaspoon salt in a shallow dish.
9. Brush the top of the fish with the remaining 1 tablespoon maple syrup.
10. Sprinkle with the cracker mixture, pressing to adhere.

11. Place the fish in the baking pan next to the carrots.

12. Lightly coat the top of the fish with cooking spray.

13. Bake for 10 to 15 minutes more or until the fish flakes easily when tested with a fork and the carrots are tender.

14. To serve, divide the carrots among dinner plates and sprinkle with the remaining 2 teaspoons pumpkin seeds.

15. Top with the salmon.

25. Vegan Cauliflower Fettuccine Alfredo with Kale

Nutritional facts: Kcal - 74, carbs - 15g, protein - 6.5g, fat - 1.5g

Ingredients: 6 servings

- ½ cup fresh whole-wheat breadcrumbs, toasted
- 1 tablespoon chopped fresh parsley
- ½ teaspoon grated lemon zest
- 4 cups cauliflower florets (1 small head)
- 1 cup raw cashews
- 8 ounces whole-wheat fettuccine
- 4 cups lightly packed thinly sliced kale
- 3 tablespoons lemon juice
- 2 tablespoons white miso
- 2 teaspoons garlic powder
- 2 teaspoons onion powder
- ¾ teaspoon salt
- 1 cup water

DIRECTIONS:

1. Put large pot of water on to boil.

2. Combine breadcrumbs, parsley and lemon zest in a small bowl.

3. Set aside.

4. Add cauliflower and cashews to the boiling water; cook until the cauliflower is very tender, about 15 minutes.

5. Using a slotted spoon, transfer cauliflower and cashews to a blender.

6. Add pasta to the boiling water and cook, stirring occasionally, for 10 minutes.

7. Add kale and cook until the pasta is just tender, about 1 minute more.

8. Drain; return the pasta and kale to the pot.

9. Add lemon juice, miso, garlic powder, onion powder, salt and 1 cup water to the blender; process until smooth.

10. Add the sauce to the pasta and stir until well coated.

11. Serve topped with the breadcrumb mixture.

26. Curried Sweet Potato & Peanut Soup

Nutritional facts: Kcal - 295, carbs - 25g, protein - 29.5g, fat - 2.9g

In this flavorful soup recipe, sweet potatoes simmer in a quick coconut curry, resulting in a creamy, thick broth punctuated by notes of garlic and ginger. We love peanuts for their inexpensive price and versatile flavor. They're also a great source of protein—1 ounce has 7 grams.

Ingredients: 6 servings

- 2 tablespoons canola oil
- 1½ cups diced yellow onion
- 1 tablespoon minced garlic
- 1 tablespoon minced fresh ginger
- 4 teaspoons red curry paste
- 1 serrano chile, ribs and seeds removed, minced
- 1 pound sweet potatoes, peeled and cubed (½-inch pieces)

- 3 cups water1 cup "lite" coconut milk
- ¾ cup unsalted dry-roasted peanuts
- 1 (15 ounce) can white beans, rinsed
- ¾ teaspoon salt¼ teaspoon ground pepper
- ¼ cup chopped fresh cilantro
- 2 tablespoons lime juice
- ¼ cup unsalted roasted pumpkin seeds
- Lime wedges

DIRECTIONS:

1. Heat oil in a large pot over medium-high heat.
2. Add onion and cook, stirring often, until softened and translucent, about 4 minutes.
3. Stir in garlic, ginger, curry paste, and serrano; cook, stirring, for 1 minute.
4. Stir in sweet potatoes and water; bring to a boil.
5. Reduce heat to medium-low and simmer, partially covered, until the sweet potatoes are soft, 10 to 12 minutes.
6. Transfer half of the soup to a blender, along with coconut milk and peanuts; puree. (Use caution when pureeing hot liquids.)
7. Return to the pot with the remaining soup.
8. Stir in beans, salt, and pepper; heat through.
9. Remove from the heat.

10. Stir in cilantro and lime juice.

11. Serve with pumpkin seeds and lime wedges.

Tip: You can find red curry paste in the Asian section of many grocery stores, packaged in a small glass jar.

To make ahead: Refrigerate soup for up to 3 days. Reheat before serving.

27. Spinach & Strawberry Salad with Poppy Seed Dressing

Nutritional facts: Kcal - 65, carbs - 14.8g, protein - 6g, fat - 1g

Homemade poppy seed dressing pairs beautifully with tender spinach, crunchy almonds and juicy berries for a fantastically refreshing and easy spring salad. To make ahead, whisk dressing, combine salad ingredients and store separately. Toss the salad with the dressing just before serving. To make it a complete meal, top with grilled chicken or shrimp.

Ingredients: 4 servings

- 2½ tablespoons mayonnaise
- 1½ tablespoons cider vinegar
- 1 tablespoon extra-virgin olive oil
- 1 teaspoon poppy seeds
- 1 teaspoon sugar¼ teaspoon salt
- ¼ teaspoon ground pepper
- 1 (5 ounce) package baby spinach

- 1 cup sliced strawberries
- ¼ cup toasted sliced almonds

DIRECTIONS:

1. Whisk mayonnaise, vinegar, oil, poppy seeds, sugar, salt and pepper in a large bowl.
2. Add spinach and strawberries and toss to coat.
3. Sprinkle with almonds.

28. Slow-Cooked Pork Tacos with Chipotle Aioli

Nutritional facts: Kcal - 250, carbs - 38.2g, protein - 17.7g, fat - 6.3g

Follow this pork taco recipe as is to serve four and you'll have enough shredded pork leftover to make it again next week. It's so good, however, that we recommend doubling the rest of the ingredients and inviting over four more friends to enjoy everything right away!

Ingredients: 4 servings

- 1 (2 to 2½ pound) boneless pork sirloin roast
- 3 tablespoons reduced-sodium taco seasoning mix
- 1 (14.5 ounce) can no-salt-added diced tomatoes, undrained
- 1 cup shredded romaine lettuce
- 1 cup chopped mango
- ⅔ cup thin bite-size strips, peeled jicama
- ½ cup light mayonnaise2 tablespoons lime juice

- 2 cloves garlic, minced
- ½ to 1 teaspoon finely chopped canned chipotle pepper in adobo sauce
- 8 (6 inch) corn tortillas, warmed
- ¼ cup coarsely chopped fresh cilantro

DIRECTIONS:

Prep: 40 m

Ready In: 4 h 10 m

1. Trim fat from roast.
2. Sprinkle with taco seasoning mix; rub in with your fingers.
3. Place the roast in a 3½- or 4-quart slow cooker.
4. Add undrained tomatoes; cover and cook on Low for 7 to 8 hours or on High for 3½ to 4 hours.
5. Remove the roast, reserving cooking liquid.
6. Shred the meat using two forks.
7. Toss the meat with enough cooking liquid to moisten.
8. Set half of the meat aside (about 2½ cups) and place the remainder in an airtight container for later use.

9. Combine lettuce, mango, and jicama in a medium bowl.

10. For chipotle aioli, combine mayonnaise, lime juice, garlic, and chipotle pepper in a small bowl.

11. Serve the shredded meat, the lettuce mixture, and the chipotle aioli in tortillas.

12. Sprinkle with cilantro.

Tips: If desired, substitute ¼ teaspoon ground chipotle chile pepper for the canned chipotle pepper.

Leftover shredded meat can be stored in an airtight container in the refrigerator up to 3 days or freezer for up to 3 months.

Equipment: 3½- or 4-quart slow cooker

29. Tofu & Snow Pea Stir-Fry with Peanut Sauce

Nutritional facts: Kcal - 175, carbs - 15.5g, protein - 2.2g, fat - 5.3g

A fast dinner recipe perfect for busy weeknights, this easy stir-fry recipe will quickly become a favorite. To save time, use precooked rice or cook rice a day ahead.

Ingredients: 4 servings

- ⅓ cup unsalted natural peanut butter
- 3 tablespoons rice vinegar
- 2 tablespoons low sodium soy sauce
- 2 teaspoons brown sugar (see Tip)
- 2 teaspoons hot sauce, such as Sriracha
- 1 (14 ounce) package extra-firm or firm tofu
- 4 teaspoons canola oil, divided
- 1 (14 ounce) package frozen (not thawed) pepper stir-fry vegetables
- 2 tablespoons finely chopped or grated fresh ginger

- 3 cloves garlic, minced2 cups fresh snow peas, trimmed
- 2 tablespoons water, plus more if needed
- 4 tablespoons unsalted roasted peanuts
- 2 cups cooked brown rice

DIRECTIONS:

Prep: 30 m

Ready In: 30 m

1. Combine peanut butter, vinegar, soy sauce, sugar, and hot sauce in a medium bowl; whisk until smooth.
2. Set aside.
3. Drain tofu; pat dry with a paper towel.
4. Cut into ¾-inch cubes; pat dry again.
5. Heat 2 tsp. oil in a large nonstick skillet over medium-high heat.
6. Add half the tofu and let cook, undisturbed, until lightly browned underneath, about 2 minutes.
7. Stir and continue cooking, stirring occasionally, until browned all over, 1 to 2 minutes.
8. Transfer to a plate.

9. Add 1 tsp. oil to the pan, then the remaining tofu; repeat.

10. Add the remaining 1 tsp. oil to the pan.

11. Add frozen vegetables, ginger, and garlic; stir-fry until the ginger and garlic are fragrant and the vegetables have thawed, 2 to 3 minutes.

12. Stir in snow peas.

13. Add water, cover and cook until the peas are crisp-tender, 3 to 4 minutes.

14. Push the vegetables to the edges of the pan.

15. Add the reserved peanut sauce to the center and cook, stirring, until hot, about 30 seconds.

16. Stir the vegetables into the sauce.

17. Add the reserved tofu and cook, stirring, until heated through, 30 to 60 seconds.

18. If necessary, add more water to make a creamy sauce.

19. Sprinkle each serving with 1 Tbsp. peanuts; serve with rice.

Tips: If using a sugar substitute, we recommend Splenda Brown Sugar Blend. Follow package directions for 2 tsp. equivalent.

Don't like tofu? Substitute 12 oz. boneless, skinless chicken breast or chicken tenders, cut into thin slices.

When you brown the chicken in Step 3, be sure that it is cooked through.

30. Chicken & Sun-Dried Tomato Orzo

Nutritional facts: Kcal - 182, carbs - 3.5g, protein - 37g, fat - 4.4g

Sun-dried tomatoes and Romano cheese pack a flavorful punch along with the tantalizing aroma of fresh marjoram in this rustic Italian-inspired dish. Serve with sautéed fresh spinach or steamed broccolini.

Ingredients: 4 servings

- 8 ounces orzo, preferably whole-wheat
- 1 cup water
- ½ cup chopped sun-dried tomatoes, (not oil-packed), divided
- 1 plum tomato, diced1 clove garlic, peeled
- 3 teaspoons chopped fresh marjoram, divided
- 1 tablespoon red-wine vinegar
- 2 teaspoons plus 1 tablespoon extra-virgin olive oil, divided

- 4 boneless, skinless chicken breasts, trimmed (1-1¼ pounds)
- ¼ teaspoon salt
- ¼ teaspoon freshly ground pepper
- 1 9-ounce package frozen artichoke hearts, thawed
- ½ cup finely shredded Romano cheese, divided

DIRECTIONS:

1. Cook orzo in a large saucepan of boiling water until just tender, 8 to 10 minutes or according to package directions.
2. Drain and rinse.
3. Meanwhile, place 1 cup water, ¼ cup sun-dried tomatoes, plum tomato, garlic, 2 teaspoons marjoram, vinegar and 2 teaspoons oil in a blender.
4. Blend until just a few chunks remain.
5. Season chicken with salt and pepper on both sides.
6. Heat remaining 1 tablespoon oil in a large skillet over medium-high heat.
7. Add the chicken and cook, adjusting the heat as necessary to prevent burning, until golden

outside and no longer pink in the middle, 3 to 5 minutes per side.

8. Transfer to a plate; tent with foil to keep warm.

9. Pour the tomato sauce into the pan and bring to a boil.

10. Measure out ½ cup sauce to a small bowl.

11. Add the remaining ¼ cup sun-dried tomatoes to the pan along with the orzo, artichoke hearts and 6 tablespoons cheese.

12. Cook, stirring, until heated through, 1 to 2 minutes.

13. Divide among 4 plates.

14. Slice the chicken.

15. Top each portion of pasta with sliced chicken, 2 tablespoons of the reserved tomato sauce and a sprinkling of the remaining cheese and marjoram.

31. Veggie yaki udon

Ingredients:

- 1½ tbsp sesame oil
- 1 red onion, cut into thin wedges
- 160g mangetout
- 70g baby corn, halved
- 2 baby pak choi, quartered
- 3 spring onions, sliced
- 1 large garlic clove, crushed
- ½ tbsp mild curry powder
- 4 tsp low-salt soy sauce
- 300g ready-to-cook udon noodles
- 1 tbsp pickled sushi ginger, chopped, plus 2 tbsp of the brine

Directions:

1. Heat the oil in a non-stick frying pan or wok over a high heat. Add the onion and fry for 5 mins. Stir in the mangetout, corn, pak choi and spring onions and cook for 5 mins more. Add the garlic,

curry powder and soy sauce, and cook for another minute.

2. Add the udon noodles along with the ginger and reserved brine and stir in 2-3 tbsp hot water until the noodles are heated through.

3. Divide between bowls and serve.

Nutritional facts: 365 calories, 9g fat, 15g protein, 51g carbs

32. Roasted red pepper & tomato soup with ricotta

Ingredients:

- 400g tomatoes, halved
- 1 red onion, quartered
- 2 Romano peppers, roughly chopped
- 2 tbsp good quality olive oil
- 2 garlic cloves bashed in their skins
- few thyme sprigs
- 1 tbsp red wine vinegar
- 2 tbsp ricotta
- few basil leaves
- 1 tbsp mixed seeds, toasted
- bread, to serve

Directions:

- Heat oven to 200C.
- Put the tomatoes, onion and peppers in a roasting tin, toss with the oil and season. Nestle in the garlic and thyme sprigs, then roast for 25-

30 mins until all the veg has softened and slightly caramelised.

- Squeeze the garlic cloves out of their skins into the tin, strip the leaves off the thyme and discard the stalks and garlic skins.
- Mix the vinegar into the tin then blend everything in a bullet blender or using a stick blender, adding enough water to loosen to your preferred consistency (we used around 150ml).
- Reheat the soup if necessary, taste for seasoning, then spoon into two bowls and top each with a spoonful of ricotta, a few basil leaves, the seeds and a drizzle of oil. Serve with bread for dunking.

Nutritional facts: 300 calories, 19g fat, 8g protein, 22g carbs

33. Veggie Okonomiyaki

Ingredients:

- 3 large eggs
- 50g plain flour
- 50ml milk
- 4 spring onion, trimmed and sliced
- 1 pak choi, sliced
- 200g Savoy cabbage, shredded
- 1 red chilli, deseeded and finely chopped, plus extra to serve
- ½ tbsp low-salt soy sauce
- ½ tbsp rapeseed oil
- 1 heaped tbsp low-fat mayonnaise
- ½ lime, juiced
- sushi ginger, to serve (optional)
- wasabi, to serve (optional)

Directions:

1. Whisk together the eggs, flour and milk until smooth.

2. Add half the spring onions, the pak choi, cabbage, chili and soy sauce. Heat the oil in a small frying pan and pour in the batter.

3. Cook, covered, over a medium heat for 7-8 mins.

4. Flip the okonomiyaki into a second frying pan, then return it to the heat and cook for a further 7-8 mins until a skewer inserted into it comes out clean.

5. Mix the mayonnaise and lime juice together in a small bowl.

6. Transfer the okonomiyaki to a plate, then drizzle over the lime mayo and top with the extra chilli and spring onion and the sushi ginger, if using.

7. Serve with the wasabi on the side, if you like.

Nutritional facts: 310 calories, 15g fat, 15g protein, 29g carbs

34. Spicy 'vedgeree'

Ingredients:

- 350g long grain brown rice
- 150g green beans, trimmed and halved
- 4 medium eggs
- 2 tbsp olive oil
- 2 onions, sliced
- 2 garlic cloves, crushed
- 2 heaped tbsp medium curry powder
- 1 tsp ground turmeric
- 2 bay leaves
- 200g spinach
- 100g cherry tomatoes, halved
- ½ small bunch coriande, chopped
- 1 green chilli, sliced
- 1 lemon, cut into wedges

Directions:

1. Rinse the rice under cold running water, rubbing with your fingers to remove any excess

starch. Cook following pack instructions, then drain well.

2. Bring another pan of water to a simmer. Cook the green beans for 2 mins, then transfer to a bowl with a slotted spoon and set aside. Boil the eggs in the pan for 7 mins, then drain and transfer to a bowl of cold water to cool.

3. Meanwhile, heat the oil in a large frying pan over a medium heat. Fry the onions for 10-15 mins until golden. Add the garlic, curry powder, turmeric and bay leaves and cook for 1 min more. Stir in the spinach, tomatoes and a splash of water and cook for another 5 mins until the spinach has wilted.

4. Fold the cooked rice and green beans through the spinach mixture and cook for a few minutes until the rice is warmed through. Drain and gently peel the eggs, then slice in half.

5. Top the rice mixture with the eggs, coriander and chilli. Serve the vedgeree with the lemon wedges on the side for squeezing over.

Nutritional facts: 500 calories, 14g fat, 20g protein, 70g carbs

35. Artichoke & Aubergine rice

Ingredients:

- 60ml olive oil
- 2 aubergine, cut into chunks
- 1 large onion, finely chopped
- 2 garlic cloves, crushed
- small pack parsley, leaves picked, stalks finely chopped
- 2 tsp smoked paprika
- 2 tsp turmeric
- 400g paella rice
- 1 ½l Kallo vegetable stock
- 2 x 175g packs chargrilled artichokes
- 2 lemons 1 juiced, 1 cut into wedges to serve

Directions:

1. Heat 2 tbsp of the oil in a large non-stick frying pan or paella pan.
2. Fry the aubergines until nicely coloured on all sides (add another tbsp of oil if the aubergine

begins catching too much), then remove and set aside.

3. Add another tbsp of oil to the pan and lightly fry the onion for 2-3 mins or until softened.

4. Add the garlic and parsley stalks, cook for a few mins more, then stir in the spices and rice until everything is well coated.

5. Heat for 2 mins, add half the stock and cook, uncovered, over a medium heat for 20 mins, stirring occasionally to prevent it from sticking.

6. Nestle the aubergine and artichokes into the mixture, pour over the rest of the stock and cook for 20 mins more or until the rice is cooked through.

7. Chop the parsley leaves, stir through with the lemon juice and season well.

8. Bring the whole pan to the table and spoon into bowls, with the lemon wedges on the side.

Nutritional facts: 430 calories, 16g fat, 8g protein, 58g carbs

36. Creamy tomato risotto

Ingredients:

- 400g can chopped tomato
- 1l vegetable stock
- knob of butter
- 1 tbsp olive oil
- 1 onion, finely chopped
- 2 garlic cloves, finely chopped
- 1 rosemary sprig, finely chopped
- 250g risotto rice
- 300g cherry tomato, halved
- small pack basil, roughly torn
- 4 tbsp grated parmesan

Directions:

1. Tip the chopped tomatoes and half the stock into a food processor and pulse until smooth. Pour into a saucepan with the remaining stock, bring to a gentle simmer and keep over a low heat.

2. Meanwhile, place the butter and oil in the base of a large saucepan and heat gently until the butter has melted. Add the onion and gently cook for 6-8 mins until softened. Stir in the garlic and rosemary, then cook for 1 min more. Add the rice and cook, stirring, for 1 min.

3. Start adding the hot stock and tomato mixture about a quarter at a time. Let the risotto cook, stirring often, adding more stock as it is absorbed. After you have added half the stock, add the cherry tomatoes. After 20-25 mins, the rice should be creamy and tender, the cherry tomatoes softened and all of the stock should be used up.

4. Cover and leave for 1 min, then stir in the basil. Serve sprinkled with Parmesan and a good grinding of black pepper.

Nutritional facts: 380 calories, 10g fat, 13g protein, 61g carbs

37. Italian borlotti bean, pumpkin & farro soup

Ingredients:

- 4 tbsp extra virgin olive oil, plus extra to serve
- 1 onion, finely chopped
- 1 celery stick, cut into chunks
- 750g pumpkin or squash, peeled, deseeded and cut into small chunks
- 1 carrot, peeled and cut into chunks
- 3 garlic cloves, chopped
- 3 tbsp tomato purée
- 1.2l chicken stock or vegetable stock
- 75g farro or mixed grains (such as barley or spelt)
- 50-80g parmesan rinds or vegetarian alternative (optional), plus a few shavings to serve
- 400g can borlotti beans, drained
- 2 handfuls baby spinach
- 2 tbsp chopped parsley or 8 whole sage leaves

Directions:

1. Heat the oil in a heavy-bottomed saucepan. Add the onion, celery, pumpkin or squash and carrot and cook until the vegetables have some colour. Add a splash of water and some seasoning, then cover the pan and let the vegetables cook over a very low heat for 5 mins.

2. Add the garlic and cook for another couple of mins, then add the tomato purée, stock, mixed grains, parmesan rinds, if using, and some seasoning. Simmer for about 15 mins (or until the grains are cooked), adding the beans for the final 5 mins. In the last few mins, add the spinach, then taste for seasoning.

3. If you want to use sage, fry the leaves whole in a little olive oil before adding to the soup. If you prefer to use parsley, you can just add it directly to the soup. Serve with shavings of parmesan and a drizzle of extra virgin olive oil on top of each bowlful. Remove the parmesan rinds and serve.

Nutritional facts: 258 calories, 11g fat, 15g protein, 21g carbs

38. Linguine with avocado, tomato & lime

Ingredients:

- 115g wholemeal linguine
- 1 lime, zested and juiced
- 1 avocado, stoned, peeled, and chopped
- 2 large ripe tomatoes, chopped
- ½ pack fresh coriander, chopped
- 1 red onion, finely chopped
- 1 red chilli, deseeded and finely chopped (optional)

Directions:

1. Cook the pasta according to pack instructions – about 10 mins. Meanwhile, put the lime juice and zest in a medium bowl with the avocado, tomatoes, coriander, onion and chilli, if using, and mix well.

2. Drain the pasta, toss into the bowl and mix well. Serve straight away while still warm, or cold.

Nutritional facts: 450 calories, 20g fat, 11g protein, 49g carbs.

39. Egyptian egg salad

Ingredients:

- 2 large eggs
- 1 lemon, juiced
- 1 tbsp tahini
- 1 tbsp rapeseed oil
- 1 red onion, chopped
- 3 large garlic cloves, finely chopped
- 1 tsp ground cumin
- ½ tsp cumin seeds
- 400g can borlotti or fava beans, juice reserved
- 2 Little Gem lettuces cut into wedges
- 2 tomatoes, cut into wedges
- sprinkling of dried chilli flakes and roughly chopped flat-leaf parsley, optional

Directions:

1. Bring a pan of water to the boil, lower in the eggs and boil for 8 mins. Drain and run under the cold tap to cool them a little, then peel and

halve. Meanwhile, mix 1 tbsp lemon juice and 3 tbsp water with the tahini to make a dressing.

2. Heat the oil and fry the onion and garlic for 5 mins to soften them. Add the ground cumin and seeds, stir briefly then add the beans and lightly crush some of them as you heat them, adding some of the juice from the can to get a nice creamy consistency but keeping whole beans, too. Taste and add lemon juice and just a little seasoning if you need to.

3. Spoon the beans on to plates with the lettuce, then add the eggs and tomatoes, with the tahini dressing, chilli and parsley, if using.

Nutritional facts: 260 calories, 12g fat, 11g protein, 17g carbs

40. Guacamole & mango salad with black beans

Ingredients:

- 1 lime, zested and juiced
- 1 small mango, stoned, peeled and chopped
- 1 small avocado, stoned, peeled and chopped
- 100g cherry tomatoes, halved
- 1 red chilli, deseeded and chopped
- 1 red onion, chopped
- ½ small pack coriander, chopped
- 400g can black beans, drained and rinsed

Directions:

- Put the lime zest and juice, mango, avocado, tomatoes, chilli and onion in a bowl, stir through the coriander and beans.

Nutritional facts: 340 calories, 15g fat, 11g protein, 33g carbs

41. Mushroom baked eggs with squished tomatoes

Ingredients:

- 2 large flat mushrooms (about 85g each), stalks removed and chopped
- rapeseed oil, for brushing
- ½ garlic clove, grated (optional)
- a few thyme leaves
- 2 tomatoes, halved
- 2 large eggs
- 2 handfuls rocket

Directions:

1. Heat oven to 200C
2. Brush the mushrooms with a little oil and the garlic (if using). Place the mushrooms in two very lightly greased gratin dishes, bottom-side up, and season lightly with pepper.
3. Top with the chopped stalks and thyme, cover with foil and bake for 20 mins.

4. Remove the foil, add the tomatoes to the dishes and break an egg carefully onto each of the mushrooms. Season and add a little more thyme, if you like. Return to the oven for 10-12 mins or until the eggs are set but the yolks are still runny. Top with the rocket and eat straight from the dishes.

Nutritional facts: 150 calories, 8g fat, 12g protein, 5g carbs

42. Healthy pasta primavera

Ingredients:

- 75g young broad beans (use frozen if you can't get fresh)
- 2 x 100g pack asparagus tips
- 170g peas (use frozen if you can't get fresh)
- 350g spaghetti or tagliatelle
- 175g pack baby leeks, trimmed and sliced
- 1 tbsp olive oil, plus extra to serve
- 1 tbsp butter
- 200ml tub fromage frais or creme fraiche
- handful fresh chopped herbs (we used mint, parsley and chives)
- parmesan (or vegetarian alternative), shaved, to serve

Directions:

- Bring a pan of salted water to the boil and put a steamer (or colander) over the water. Steam the beans, asparagus and peas until just tender, then set aside. Boil the pasta following pack instructions.

- Meanwhile, fry the leeks gently in the oil and butter for 5 mins or until soft. Add the fromage frais to the leeks and very gently warm through, stirring constantly to ensure it doesn't split. Add the herbs and steamed vegetables with a splash of pasta water to loosen.

- Drain the pasta and stir into the sauce. Adjust the seasoning, then serve scattered with the cheese and drizzled with a little extra olive oil.

Nutritional facts: 475 calories, 9g fat, 20g protein, 75g carbs

43. Pea & broad bean shakshuka

Ingredients:

- 1 bunch asparagus spears
- 200g sprouting broccoli
- 2 tbsp olive oil
- 2 spring onion, finely sliced
- 2 tsp cumin seeds
- large pinch cayenne pepper, plus extra to serve
- 4 ripe tomatoes, chopped
- 1 small pack parsle, finely chopped
- 50g shelled peas
- 50g podded broad beans
- 4 large eggs
- 50g pea shoots
- Greek yogurt and flatbreads, to serve

Directions:

1. Trim or snap the woody ends of the asparagus and finely slice the spears, leaving the tips and about 2cm at the top intact.

2. Finely slice the broccoli in the same way, leaving the heads and about 2cm of stalk intact. Heat the oil in a frying pan.

3. Add the spring onions, sliced asparagus and sliced broccoli, and fry gently until the veg softens a little, then add the cumin seeds, cayenne, tomatoes (with their juices), parsley and plenty of seasoning, and stir.

4. Cover with a lid and cook for 5 mins to make a base sauce, then add the asparagus spears, broccoli heads, peas and broad beans, cover again and cook for 2 mins.

5. Make 4 dips in the mixture. Break an egg into each dip, arrange half the pea shoots around the eggs, season well, cover with a lid and cook until the egg whites are just set.

6. Serve with the rest of the pea shoots, a spoonful of yogurt and some flatbreads, and sprinkle over another pinch of cayenne, if you like.

Nutritional facts: 200 calories, 12g fat, 13g protein, 7g carbs

44. Crispy Falafel

Ingredients:

- ¼ cup + 1 tablespoon extra-virgin olive oil
- 1 cup dried (uncooked/raw) chickpeas, rinsed, picked over and soaked for at least 4 hours and up to 24 hours in the refrigerator
- ½ cup roughly chopped red onion (about ½ small red onion)
- ½ cup packed fresh parsley (mostly leaves but small stems are ok)
- ½ cup packed fresh cilantro (mostly leaves but small stems are ok)
- 4 cloves garlic, quartered
- 1 teaspoon fine sea salt
- ½ teaspoon (about 25 twists) freshly ground black pepper
- ½ teaspoon ground cumin
- ¼ teaspoon ground cinnamon

Directions:

1. With an oven rack in the middle position, preheat oven to 375 degrees Fahrenheit. Pour ¼ cup of the olive oil into a large, rimmed baking sheet and turn until the pan is evenly coated.

2. In a food processor, combine the soaked and drained chickpeas, onion, parsley, cilantro, garlic, salt, pepper, cumin, cinnamon, and the remaining 1 tablespoon of olive oil. Process until smooth, about 1 minute.

3. Using your hands, scoop out about 2 tablespoons of the mixture at a time. Shape the falafel into small patties, about 2 inches wide and ½ inch thick. Place each falafel on your oiled pan.

4. Bake for 25 to 30 minutes, carefully flipping the falafels halfway through baking, until the falafels are deeply golden on both sides. These falafels keep well in the refrigerator for up to 4 days or in the freezer for several months.

Nutritional facts: 310 calories, 11g fat, 17g protein, 24g carbs

45. Epic Vegetarian Tacos

Ingredients:

- Quick-pickled onions
- Creamy avocado dip
- Easy refried beans
- 8 corn tortillas
- Salsa verde
- Shredded green cabbage (for extra crunch)
- Crumbled Cotija or feta cheese
- Chopped fresh cilantro
- Lime wedges

Directions:

1. Prepare the onions, avocado dip, and beans as directed, in that order.
2. Once they're ready, warm the tortillas in a large skillet over medium heat in batches, flipping to warm each side. Alternatively, you can warm them directly over a low flame on a gas range.

Stack the warmed tortillas on a plate and cover with a tea towel to keep warm.

3. To assemble the tacos, spread refried beans down the center of each tortilla. Top with avocado dip and onions (for reference, I used all of the beans and about half of the avocado dip and onions). Finish the tacos with garnishes of your choice, and serve immediately.

4. Leftover components are best served separately; reheat the tortillas and beans before serving. Leftover pickled onions and avocado dip are great on quesadillas, nachos or tortilla chips, sandwiches, etc...

Nutritional facts: 155 calories, 9g fat, 18g protein, 38g carbs

46. Spaghetti Squash Burrito Bowls

Ingredients:

- 2 cups purple cabbage, thinly sliced and roughly chopped into 2-inch long pieces
- 1 can (15 ounces) black beans, rinsed and drained
- 1 red bell pepper, chopped
- ⅓ cup chopped green onions, both green and white parts
- ⅓ cup chopped fresh cilantro
- 2 to 3 tablespoons fresh lime juice, to taste
- 1 teaspoon olive oil
- ¼ teaspoon salt
- ¾ cup mild salsa verde, either homemade or store-bought
- 1 ripe avocado, diced
- ⅓ cup fresh cilantro (a few stems are ok)
- 1 tablespoon fresh lime juice
- 1 medium garlic clove, roughly chopped

Directions:

1. To roast the spaghetti squash: Preheat the oven to 400 degrees Fahrenheit and line a large baking sheet with parchment paper for easy clean-up. On the baking sheet, drizzle the halved spaghetti squash with olive oil. Rub the olive oil all over each of the halves, adding more if necessary.

2. Sprinkle the insides of the squash with freshly ground black pepper and salt. Turn them over so the insides are facing down. Roast for 40 to 60 minutes, until the flesh is easily pierced through with a fork.

3. Meanwhile, to assemble the slaw: In a medium mixing bowl, combine the cabbage, black beans, bell pepper, green onion, cilantro, lime juice, olive oil and salt. Toss to combine and set aside to marinate.

4. To make the salsa verde: In the bowl of a blender or food processor, combine the avocado, salsa verde, cilantro, lime juice and garlic. Blend until smooth, pausing to scrape down the sides as necessary.

5. To assemble, first use a fork to separate and fluff up the flesh of the spaghetti squash. Then divide the slaw into each of the spaghetti squash "bowls," and add a big dollop of avocado salsa verde. Finish the bowls with another sprinkle of pepper, cilantro and optional crumbled feta or pepitas.

Nutritional facts: 245 calories, 8g fat, 21g protein, 64g carbs

47. Roasted Cauliflower and Farro Salad with Feta and Avocado

---

Ingredients:

- 1 large head cauliflower (about 2 pounds), cut into bite-sized florets
- 2 tablespoons extra-virgin olive oil
- ¼ teaspoon red pepper flakes (scale back or omit if sensitive to spice)
- ¼ teaspoon fine sea salt
- 1 cup uncooked farro, rinsed
- 2 teaspoons extra-virgin olive oil
- 2 cloves garlic, pressed or minced
- ¼ teaspoon fine sea salt

Directions:

1. To roast the cauliflower: Preheat the oven to 425 degrees Fahrenheit. Toss the cauliflower florets with the olive oil, red pepper flakes and salt, and arrange it in an even layer across the pan. Roast for 25 to 35 minutes, tossing halfway, until the

cauliflower is tender and deeply golden on the edges.

2. To cook the farro: In a medium saucepan, combine the rinsed farro with at least three cups water (enough water to cover the farro by a couple of inches). Bring the water to a boil, then reduce the heat to a gentle simmer, and cook until the farro is tender to the bite but still pleasantly chewy. (Pearled farro will take around 15 minutes; unprocessed farro will take 25 to 40 minutes.) Drain off the excess water and mix in the olive oil, garlic and salt. Set aside.

3. In a large serving bowl, toss together the roasted cauliflower, cooked farro, olives, sun-dried tomatoes, feta and lemon juice. Taste and season with additional salt and pepper if necessary.

4. Divide the avocado and greens between four dinner plates. Top with a generous amount of the cauliflower and farro salad. Finish the plates with an extra squeeze of lemon juice or drizzle of olive oil, if desired. Serve promptly.

Nutritional facts: 385 calories, 12g fat, 19g protein, 65g carbs

Conclusion

As we conclude this guide, we must remember that the intermittent fasting is a diet plan designed to involves a period of fasting followed by a period of non-fasting. By changing your eating habits according to this diet, you will lower your sugar intake which will then cause your blood pressure to be reduced. IF is not focused on what you can eat, but how and when you can eat.

You will see a difference within two weeks and your weight can drop by as soon as you expect after only a short period of time. So, as we begin the diet, let us give you more basic tips about IF if you are a woman above 50. There really is no reason to wait for months to start improving your health. This diet can help to prevent a number of illnesses, including cancer, diabetes, stroke and even heart disease.

FOODS TO EAT

You can have certain fats and sweets, but they need to be limited. Your diet needs to consist of mainly whole grains (6-8 servings per day), vegetables (4-5 servings per day), fruits (4-5 servings per day) and low-fat dairy products (2-3 servings per day) to be effective.

Lean meat, poultry and fish need to be limited to a maximum of 6 servings per day. Nuts, legumes and seeds should be limited to 4-5 servings per week, and then there is fat and oils, which are allowed, but should be limited to 2 servings per day.

If you are wondering about the sweet stuff, then wonder no more! You are not allowed to take sweets in the IF diet, but if really want to take them, you need to limit them to not more than 2 servings per week.

HOW MUCH IS A SINGLE SERVING?

Here are some examples of serving sizes to get you going on the road to better health:

GRAINS - One slice of bread, 1/2 cup of cooked pasta, cereal and rice, or 1 ounce of dry cereal.

VEGETABLES - One cup of leafy green veggies or 1/2 cup of cooked or raw veggies.

FRUIT - One medium fruit, 1/2 cup of canned, fresh or frozen fruit.

DAIRY - One cup of yogurt, 1 cup of skim/1% milk or1 1/2 ounces of cheese.

LEAN MEAT, FISH & POULTRY - One egg, 1 ounce of cooked lean meat or 1 ounce of canned tuna in water.

NUTS, SEEDS AND LEGUMES - 1/3 cup of nuts, 1/2 cup of cooked peas or beans, or 2 tablespoons of seeds.

FATS AND OILS - Two tablespoons of dressing, 1 teaspoon of margarine (soft) or 1 tablespoon of low-fat mayonnaise.

SWEETS - One cup of lemonade, 1/2 cup of sorbet or one tablespoon of jelly, sugar or jam.

Try to avoid most processed foods, alcohol and processed sweets where possible, but give yourself the odd treat now and then. Good luck and enjoy your dieting.

If you liked this book, recommend it and write a review, please. I'll be grateful.

Elisabeth Holland

CPSIA information can be obtained
at www.ICGtesting.com
Printed in the USA
BVHW091109090621
609092BV00003B/657